Karen Ashton
THE ESSENTIAL OILS

Copyright

All materials and contents are owned and licensed by Karen Ashton of Holistic Therapies Training. Any copying, adaption or use of any material without written permission of Holistic Therapies Training is strictly prohibited. Diagrams / images / text, unless stated otherwise, are provided for use by Karen Ashton at Holistic Therapies Training only.

Liability

Holistic Therapies Training will accept no liability to any person for any type of loss, damage whatsoever resulting from the use of the material within this book or any book published by Karen Ashton of Holistic Therapies Training.

Medical Disclaimer

It is strongly advised that you take medical advice if you or any of your clients have a health problem. Holistic Therapies Training or any book, material or qualification from Holistic Therapies Training will not qualify you to advise on any medical condition or to diagnose a condition. Alternative health care should not be taken as a substitute for any medical care.

Disclaimer

It is the readers sole responsibility to ensure they receive the correct training, sufficient for their needs and for insurance purposes, this book will only support a qualification it will not qualify you to consult with clients.

Karen Ashton
THE ESSENTIAL OILS GUIDE

All rights reserved. No part of this publication may be reproduced in any form or by any means including, scanning, photocopying, or otherwise without prior written permission of the copyright holder.

Copyright © 2019 Karen Ashton. Holistic Tutor – www.holistictherapiestraining.co.uk

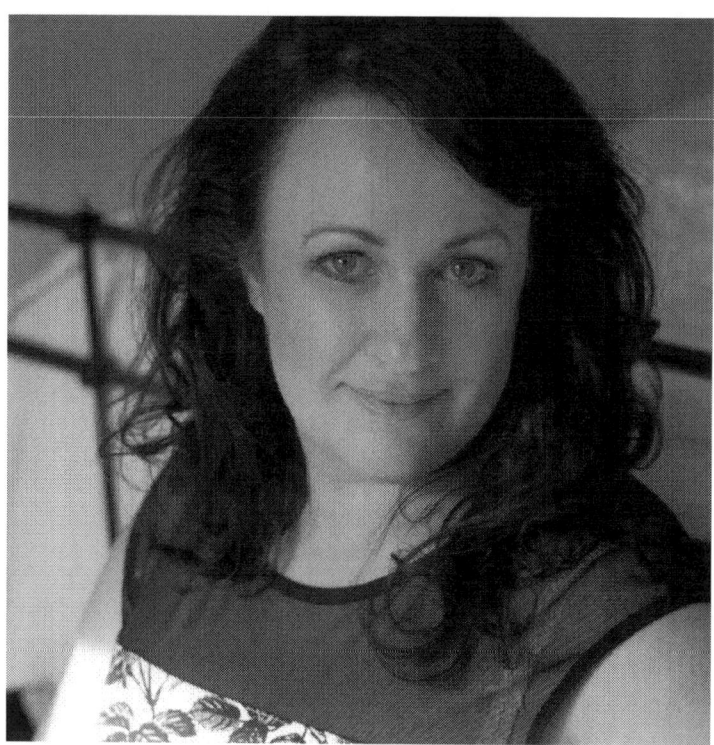

Karen Ashton
THE ESSENTIAL OILS GUIDE

Acknowledgements

The contents of this book were originally created for my level 3 aromatherapy students and the essential oil guide for my own reference as well.

This led me to wanting to share this information with others, far and wide.

I would like to thank my husband, 'the hubster', Jason for his patience in my putting together of this book and talking me into publishing it, on many occasions! It is funny how the universe works, as without having a six-week recovery period from a total hip replacement, I probably would still be only halfway through writing this book now. And thinking of a hundred and one reasons not to publish!

I would like to make a special acknowledgement to my beautiful boys, Kieran & Connor, who are my world!

An acknowledgement to my students, past & present, who have been a joy to teach, and often brings the phrase to mind, 'and they call this work?' I have spent many a day with these lovely people, making lotions and potions and experimenting with the oils. Having the fits of giggles when my husband decided to use a rather potent blend of Neroli in our diffuser for an aromatherapy training day, so myself and students, enjoyed a rather 'happy' day floating ☐

I love the aha moments that the training brings to the students and their lightbulb moments where they realise their special gifts or niche that they can bring to the industry or a piece of information I provide them about the oils.

May there be many more!

Karen Ashton
THE ESSENTIAL OILS GUIDE

Contents

Copyright 1

Acknowledgements 3

Glossary 7

Synergy 11

Adaptogen 11

Top Notes 12

Middle Notes 12

Base Notes 12

Proportions 13

Chemical constituents 14

What to look for when choosing essential oils (adulteration) 17

    Factors to consider when purchasing essential oils 18

The history of Aromatherapy 18

The benefits of Aromatherapy 20

Taxonomy, nomenclature, structure and function of plants: 21

Characteristics of essential oils (essences): 23

Methods of extraction (essences): 25

Methods of use and application: 26

Other aromatherapy mediums and sources: 27

Basil 30

Karen Ashton
THE ESSENTIAL OILS GUIDE

Benzoin 35

Bergamot 39

Black Pepper 44

Cedarwood Atlas 50

Chamomile German / Chamomile Roman 54

Clary Sage 58

Cypress 61

Eucalyptus 65

Fennel 71

Frankincense 75

Geranium 80

Ginger 85

Ginger & Lemon for joint pain 89

Grapefruit 91

Jasmine 96

Juniper 100

Lavandin 104

Lavender 108

Lavender Spike 113

Lemon 117

Lemongrass 121

Mandarin 125

Marjoram 129

Karen Ashton
THE ESSENTIAL OILS GUIDE

Myrrh 133

Neroli 137

Orange (Sweet) 141

Patchouli 145

Peppermint 150

Petitgrain 155

Rose 158

Rosemary 162

Sandalwood 167

Tea Tree 171

Thyme 176

Vetivert 181

Ylang Ylang 185

Safety Guidelines 189

Objectives chart 193

Skin type chart 195

Skin condition chart 196

Top, Middle, Base Note Chart 197

How my journey started 198

About the author 207

Karen Ashton
THE ESSENTIAL OILS GUIDE

Introduction

This essential oil guide has been compiled, primarily for my students completing their VTCT level 3 Aromatherapy qualification, to help them with their selection of essential oils for their case studies, but also for many people to benefit from, whether for their own use or for clients.

Aromatherapy has been a passion of mine for decades, but I finally achieved my career change in 2003 to become, initially an aromatherapist & to set up an online shop selling essential oils and aromatherapy products. Followed on by further therapies to become a holistic therapist. I qualified as a further education teacher in 2007 and Holistic Therapies Training was launched. Aromatherapy is one of my favourite therapies to teach to my students and what I love the most about this therapy is there is no end to what you can learn about using essential oils.

I hope this handbook will prove useful to you whether for home use, clients or students.

This handbook includes the essential oils covered in the VTCT Level 3 Diploma in Aromatherapy.

Karen Ashton
Holistic Tutor
www.holistictherapiestraining.co.uk

Karen Ashton
THE ESSENTIAL OILS GUIDE

Glossary

- **Analgesic – Relieves Pain**
- Anaphrodisiac – Reduces sexual desire
- Anaesthetic – Pain reliever, loss of sensation
- Antacid – Balances the acidity in the body
- **Anti-allergenic - Treating allergies**
- **Antibacterial/bactericidal – Helps to kill bacteria**
- Anticoagulant – Prevents or delays blood from clotting
- **Anticonvulsive – Helps to treat epilepsy**
- **antidepressant – Uplifting, alleviates depression**
- Antidontalgic – Relieves toothache
- **Anti-inflammatory – Alleviates inflammation**
- **Antiemetic – Helps to prevent vomiting and nausea**
- **Antimicrobial – Destroys or resists pathogenic micro-organisms**
- Antineuralgic – Reduces nerve pain
- **Antiphlogistic – Helps to prevent inflammation**
- Antiputrefactive – Delays composition of animal / vegetables
- **Antipruritic – Relieves itching**
- **Antirheumatic – Helps to slow down the process of rheumatism**
- Antisclerotic – Prevents hardening of tissue
- Antiscorbutic – Aids to prevent scurvy

Karen Ashton
THE ESSENTIAL OILS GUIDE

- Antiseptic – Destroys and prevents the development of microbes.
- Antispasmodic – Relieves cramp, prevents or eases spasms or convulsions.
- Antisudorific – Reduces sweating
- Antivenomous – Medication to treat poisonous insect or snake bits
- Antiviral – Inhibits the growth of a virus
- Aperitif – Stimulates the appetite
- Aphrodisiac – Stimulates or increases sexual desire
- Astringent – Contracts bodily tissues and help to control infection
- Bactericide – A substance that kills bacteria
- Balsamic – An aromatic ointment for medicinal use. (Balsam comes from trees)
- Bechic – Soothing and eases coughs
- Cardiac - Good for the heart
- Carminative – Relieves flatulence
- Cephalic – Stimulates and clears the mind
- Cholagogue – Promotes discharge of bile from the system
- Cordial – Warming tonic to the heart and circulation
- Cicatrisant – Helps wounds to heal, good for scarring
- Cytophalactic – Encourages cell regeneration
- Decongestant – Loosens mucous
- Deodorant – Reduces odour
- Depurative – Purifies the blood

Karen Ashton
THE ESSENTIAL OILS GUIDE

- Detoxicant – Cleanses the body of impurities
- Digestive – Helps with digestion
- Disinfectant – Destroys germs
- Diuretic – Stimulates urine secretion
- Emmenagogue – Induces / assists with menstruation
- Emollient – Softening & Soothing to the skin
- Escharotic – Treats warts
- Expectorant – Aids removal of catarrh
- Febrifuge – Reduces fever
- Fungicide – Kills parasites
- Galactagogue – Increases milk supply
- Haemostatic – Stems bleeding / haemorrhaging
- Hepatic – Relating to the liver
- Hypertensive – Increases blood pressure
- Hypoglycaemia – High levels of glucose in the blood
- Hypotensive – Reduces blood pressure
- Insecticide – Repels insects
- Laxative – Treats constipation
- Nervine – Calms the nerves
- Parturient – Aids in an easier childbirth
- Prophylactic – Helps to prevent diseases
- Resolvent – Helps to rid boils & skin eruptions
- Restorative – Restores health & well-being
- Rubefacient – Increases local circulation, and creates erythema
- Sedative – Calms
- Splenetic – Helps with inflammation of the liver
- Stimulant – Uplifts and rouses the mind / body

Karen Ashton
THE ESSENTIAL OILS GUIDE

- Stomachic – Promotes the appetite and assists in digestion
- Styptic – Helps to stop bleeding
- Sudorific – Induces sweating
- Tonic – Strengthens and enlivens the body
- Uterine – A tonic to the uterus
- Vasoconstrictor – Contracts blood vessel walls
- Vermifuge – Destroys intestinal worms
- Vulnerary – Helps to heal wounds and sores

Synergy

When two or more essential oils are blended together, the chemistry of the oils combine with one another to create an entirely new substance whose properties as a whole add up to more than the sum of its individual parts, and thus creates a synergistic blend which is more powerful than using an individual oil on its own.

A harmonious blend would consist of a top, middle and base note, although it does not affect the therapeutic properties of a blend if it is not always possible to create a harmonious blend, this will depend on what oils are selected for their suitability to the client and the treatment.

Karen Ashton
THE ESSENTIAL OILS GUIDE

So, what are top, middle and base notes?

Adaptogen

Adaptogens are oils, such as lemon and lavender, which adapt to what your body needs, and adapt to that situation.

Top Notes

Essential oils that are classified as top notes normally evaporate very fast. They tend to be light, fresh and uplifting in nature and are usually inexpensive. Top notes are highly volatile, fast acting, and give the first impression of the blend. However, they do not last for long. Examples of top notes are Bergamot, Lemon, Lemongrass, Sweet Orange, Lime, Grapefruit, Eucalyptus.

Middle Notes

Middle notes usually give body to the blend and have a balancing effect. The aroma of middle notes are not always immediately evident and may take a couple of minutes to establish their scent. They are usually warm and soft fragrances. Examples of middle notes are Lavender, Geranium, Rosemary, Black Pepper, Juniper, Marjoram.

Karen Ashton
THE ESSENTIAL OILS GUIDE

Base Notes

Essential oils that are classified as base notes are normally very heavy and their fragrance is very solid. It will be present for a long time and slows down the evaporation of the other oils. These fragrances are normally intense and heady. They are normally rich and relaxing in nature and are typically the most expensive of all oils. Examples of base notes are Ylang Ylang, Sandalwood, Frankincense, Jasmine, Patchouli, Rose.

Proportions

Here are suggested blending proportions:

Massage Essential Oil	Carrier Oil	Percentage
Face Massage 1 drop	5ML	1%
Back Massage 4 – 5 drops	10ML	2% - 2 ½%
Fully Body Massage 10 – 12 drops	25ML	2% - 2 ½%
Children, Pre-Natal, & Elderly 2 drops	10ML	1%

Karen Ashton
THE ESSENTIAL OILS GUIDE

The amount of essential oil used in your blend can vary from 0.5% - 3% depending on the client's condition and their size. We adopt a 2 – 2 ½% for adults. If you use the 2 ½% method it helps by halving the amount of carrier millilitres used, for example for 10MLs of carrier oil you would use a maximum of 5 drops of carrier oil to create a 2 ½% dilution.

Chemical constituents

Chemical constituents build the 'ingredients' of the essential oil, its classification, character, odour and their individual qualities. Every essential oil will contain several constituents. Here are some descriptions of a few of the major constituents:

<u>Alcohols</u>
Alcohols are based on monoterpenes and contain ten carbon atoms. Alcohol substances in essential oils have good antiseptic and anti-viral properties as well as having uplifting qualities. Common examples include Linalool, is a major constituent of Lavender; and Citronellal, this is found in Rose, Lemon, Eucalyptus and Geranium.

Karen Ashton
THE ESSENTIAL OILS GUIDE

Terpenes
In most essential oils. Absorbs oxygen easily. Some terpenes can cause skin irritation if they contain a high portion of terpenes. They contain widely varying properties. They contain anti-viral (i.e., Lemon), anti-inflammatory & bacterial properties (i.e., chamomile), antiseptic properties (i.e., Pine).
Terpenes include:
* Monoterpenes – stimulating properties, i.e., Lemon, Bergamot, Neroli, Cypress
* Sesquiterpenes – Balancing properties i.e., Chamomile

Aldehydes
Aldehydes are most commonly found in lemon scented oils and they generally have sedating but uplifting qualities. Contained in oils such as Benzoin, Lemon, Lemongrass, Marjoram sweet.

Esters
Esters are among the most common compounds found in essential oils and they have fungicidal and sedative properties. Found in oils such as Basil, Benzoin, Bergamot, Cajeput, Chamomile, Clary Sage etc.

Ketones
Some Ketones are potentially toxic, so oils containing large quantities of this need to be treated with a degree of caution, as per the list of hazardous oils. But not all

Karen Ashton
THE ESSENTIAL OILS GUIDE

Ketones are bad, e.g., Jasmine and Sweet Fennel contain relatively benign Ketones and are helpful with problems affecting the upper respiratory tract.

Lactones
These are found mainly in expressed oils. A sub-group of lactones called 'furocoumarins' are known as photo-sensitisers contained in oils such as Grapefruit & Lemon; and 'bergapten' is the most common molecular example. E.g. Bergamot Oil.

Oxides
Oxides are commonly found in Camphoraceous oils and tend to have expectorant effects. E.g., Rosemary, Eucalyptus and Tea Tree.

Acids
This is a rare component of essential oils. They are based structurally on carboxyl group and have the chemical grouping COOH. Acids have a low volatile rate and are found in oils such as Benzoin and Geranium.

Ethers
Phenolic ethers are the most widely found ethers in essential oils with anethol found in aniseed, the only real ether of importance together with methyl chavicol found in basil and tarragon.

Karen Ashton
THE ESSENTIAL OILS GUIDE

<u>Phenols</u>
Phenols are bacterial and have a strong stimulating effect on the central nervous system. But any oil that contains large quantities of some Phenols can cause potential skin irritation. Found in oils such as Basil, Chamomile, Fennel Sweet, Jasmine etc.

What to look for when choosing essential oils (adulteration)

The shelf life of essential oils, carrier oils and massage oils can vary greatly, and their life expectancy can be influenced by many different external factors such as:

- incorrect light exposure
- heat exposure
- air exposure
- extended storage periods

When oils start the degradation process, hydrolysis (process of breaking the bonds) occurs as well as oxidation.

Unfortunately, due the widespread popularity of essential oils, there is an increased practice of adulteration, which takes on several forms:

- A very small quantity can be diluted into a spirit base.

Karen Ashton
THE ESSENTIAL OILS GUIDE

- Synthetic aromatic substances can be added, which results in fabricated oils.
- A quantity of the main chemical constituent may be added to the essential oils to 'stretch' it.
- An essential oil from cheaper plant may be added, e.g., lemon to bergamot, or citronella to Melissa.
- A substitute oil is used.
- Some of the chemical constituents may be removed, these oils are known as fractioned oils.

Factors to consider when purchasing essential oils

It is very important to buy essential oils from a reputable supplier.

The following factors should be considered when purchasing your oils:

- Quality
- Purity
- Price
- Odour
- Best before date
- Origin
- Botanical name of plant
- Safety

A reputable supplier will provide an MSDS sheet (Manufacture Safety Data Sheet) and a statement of analysis or similar.

Karen Ashton
THE ESSENTIAL OILS GUIDE

The history of Aromatherapy

Aromatherapy dates back to as far as ancient 2000 BC. Records in the bible show the use of plants and their aromatic oils both for the treatment of illnesses and for religious purposes.

The ancient Egyptians used the aromatic oils in cosmetics and the perfume was voted the favourite in the whole of the middle east.

The Greeks and Romans obtained most of their knowledge about aromatherapy from the Egyptians and used the aromatic oils in massage and daily bathing

A French cosmetic chemist named Rene- Maurice Gattefosse, in the 1920's, then discovered the healing properties of the essential oils / plant medicine while burning himself whilst making fragrances in his laboratory and discovered that the essential oil of lavender was exceptionally healing to the skin and left no scarring. This discovery then caused him to undergo extensive research into the medicinal uses of the oils, in which he discovered that it was possible for the essential oils to penetrate the skin and be carried in the blood and lymphatic system to the organs.

Karen Ashton
THE ESSENTIAL OILS GUIDE

China and India have a long history of using plants and herbs as medicine. Chinese medicine is still used today throughout the world ranging from Herbalism to Shiatsu.

In the Middle Ages, people protected themselves from infections by wearing herbal bouquets and they perfumed their homes by throwing herbs on the floor, as well as warding off infections.

In the 15th & 16th centuries, Columbus and Cortes, explorers, brought new plants back to Europe from their expeditions to the Americas. But, the use of aromatic plants became more unpopular when the Industrial Revolution hit Britain, when the production of synthetic plant oils over ruled the ancient use of pure aromatic plant oils.

A French surgeon, called Jean Valnet, established the medicinal uses of essential oils, which he used as antiseptics in the treatment of wounded soldiers during World War II.

The modern role of aromatherapy continues to validate what the ancients and history of aromatherapy has already known, that essential oils are a unique form of modern-day healing with many benefits as a complementary therapy.

Karen Ashton
THE ESSENTIAL OILS GUIDE

The benefits of Aromatherapy

- Promote homeostasis - Maintain health by encouraging the body to heal, re-balances the whole system to restore homeostasis, can help many ailments to restore health, as well as being a preventative for future illnesses.
- Deep relaxation – The massage techniques / aromatherapy treatment can bring about a state of deep relaxation for the client.
- Stress relief –The client receiving some 'me' time and the massage techniques helps to reduce physical and mental stress in the body.
- Pain relief by releasing endorphins into the body which are the body's pain killing hormones.
- Reduced muscle tension
- Increased energy levels by promoting energy flows in the body.
- Improved sense of well-being by releasing endorphins in the body to lift the mood, as well as serotonin also found in anti-depressant drugs.
- Stimulation of the body systems
- Lymphatic drainage allowing the body to rid itself of toxins
- Maintenance of good health
- Improves physical condition by improving muscle tone, blood & lymph circulation

Karen Ashton
THE ESSENTIAL OILS GUIDE

Taxonomy, nomenclature, structure and function of plants:

The huge variety of essential oils are derived from the plant kingdom and are present in a plant in special cells, and may be extracted from various parts of the plant matter, e.g. the leaves, flowers, fruit, grass, root, wood, bark, rhizome (mass of roots), gums, blossom, stem, and seeds.

They are usually present in minute quantities in comparison to the mass of the whole plant and may exist in the plant material in concentrations ranging from 0.01 to 10 %.

They are subject to several processes and can vary according to:
- Where they are grown
- The climate
- The altitude
- The soil
- The agricultural methods
- The time of harvesting

It is therefore very important that the starting material used to produce the essential oil represents the natural biochemistry of the plant, in order that an oil with the highest grade of quality may be produced.

Karen Ashton
THE ESSENTIAL OILS GUIDE

Due to their differences in distribution there are several methods of producing essential oils.

These are:
- Steam distillation
- Solvent extraction
- Expression
- Enfleurage
- Super-critical carbon dioxide extraction
- Phytonic process

Plant family – Most Aromatherapy books will state which plant family the essential oil is produced from. For example: (Sweet) Orange comes from the Ruttaceae plant family.

Chemotypes – Where an essential oil is of different chemical composition, even though they are obtained from plants which are botanically identical. They can vary from season to season and plants grown in different regions and under different conditions can produce essential oils with widely diverse characteristics.

Botany, plant biology, is the science of plants. A plant formation is a community of plant species, some of which are predominate.

Karen Ashton
THE ESSENTIAL OILS GUIDE

Characteristics of essential oils (essences):

Essential oils have many characteristics which are listed below:

- Aromatic
  Each essential oil has their own individual fragrance, and when combined and blended will create a completely different fragrance to that of the oils singly.
- Volatile
  Some oils are more volatile than others, i.e., they will evaporate quicker – e.g., citrus oils tend to evaporate quicker than other oils.
- Powerful
  It is essential to realise the power of the oils when selecting the blends. Some oils, such as clary sage, are more powerful than others and may have more of an effect on the client.
- oil soluble
  Some plant materials that make up the essential oils are oil soluble which means they will dissolve in oil, e.g. lipophilic.
- Alcohol soluble
  some plant materials that make up the essential oils are alcohol soluble which means they will dissolve in alcohol.
- Lipophilic
  Oil soluble
- Hydrophilic

An oil which is easier to dissolve in water liquid
- non-greasy
- Flammable
Essential oils are flammable, so it is important to keep them away from naked flames.

Methods of extraction (essences):

Water / Steam Distillation

Steam distillation converts the volatile liquid (the essential oils) into a vapour and then condenses the vapour back into a liquid - it is the most popular and cost-effective method in use today in producing essential oils.

Solvent Extraction

Solvent extraction is where solvents are used to coax the essential oils out of the botanical material, and various ways are also employed.

Expression

Expression is a cold pressed method of extraction, which is mostly used in the extraction of citrus essential oils.

Enfleurage

Enfleurage is the traditional method used to extract the finest quality essences from delicate flowers such as rose and jasmine which continue to generate oil after harvesting.

Super-critical carbon dioxide extraction

This is a relatively new method of extracting essential oils and uses compressed carbon dioxide at very high pressure to extract the essential oil from the plant material.

Hydro Diffusion / Percolation

When essential oils are extracted using hydro diffusion it is a type of steam distillation, and only varies in the actual way in which the steam is introduced into the still. With hydro diffusion the steam is fed in from the top onto the botanical material instead of from the bottom as in normal steam distillation.

Karen Ashton
THE ESSENTIAL OILS GUIDE

Methods of use and application:

- Add to bath water, use in shower
- Add to creams and lotions such as cleansers, moisturisers, Face Masks, salt scrubs
- Add to hydrolats to make flower waters and sprays such as room sprays and face spritz
- Used to inhale from a handkerchief or on your pillow
- Steam inhalation, nasal inhalers
- To fragrance your ironing, you can add a drop or two to the water in your iron.
- Add to an oil burner / diffuser
- Hot or cold compresses
- Shampoos, Conditioners, Deep conditioning treatments
- Foot spa
- Massages
- Soap making
- Making your own perfume

There is no end to ways in which you can use essential oils

Karen Ashton
THE ESSENTIAL OILS GUIDE

Other aromatherapy mediums and sources:

Advantages/disadvantages of:

- Wax – Can be used in paraffin wax or candle making. Disadvantage - Care needs to be taken when using in candle making as the essential oils can be highly flammable when the oil is exposed to a naked flame, also the heat may lessen the therapeutic properties of the oil by weakening the aroma. Advantages – will create an aroma to be absorbed into the skin when used in paraffin wax or to inhale when used in candle making as the flame heats the candlewax to disperse the smell.
- Creams – Essential oils can be blended into creams for the face and body and may be a preferable way of applying to the body as opposed to fixed / carrier oils. Advantages – less oily, can be used daily in skin care regime. Disadvantage – if the cream is blended for future use the cream would need to be stored in a secure pot as the oils may evaporate and become volatile.
- Lotions – The same as creams above.
- Gels – Can be used as an ointment such as antiseptic. Again, the disadvantage is if it is blended for future use the cream would need to

be stored in a secure pot as the oils may evaporate and become volatile
- Water – To add a few drops to water in the bath or in an oil burner can create the desired therapeutic effect either by inhalation or absorption into the skin. The disadvantage of using in bath water is that oil does not dissolve into water very well so can sit on the surface of the water causing irritation to the skin, so it is important to dilute the oils correctly in a fixed oil or full fat milk.
- Air – The oils can be heated in an oil burner to disperse into the air where you can inhale the aroma and the therapeutic properties. The disadvantage is that this cannot have such a quick effect as absorption as the aroma is not directed at you or the client, unlike in a steamer, as the aroma will disperse into the air.
- Clay – Oils can be mixed into clay and applied as a face mask, so the therapeutic properties absorb directly into the skin on the face.
- Hydrolats – These can be used as a facial toner or iron water. It is important to use distilled water when using it in the iron.
- shea butter – Ideal for dry skin as the shea butter will give moisture as well as the therapeutic properties of the oils used.
- cocoa butter – as above but with the added advantage of being ideal for skin with stretch marks or wrinkles.

Karen Ashton
THE ESSENTIAL OILS GUIDE

N.B.

Aromatherapy or any complementary therapies should not substitute medical care. If you think you have a medical condition you should always get this confirmed by your GP or similar professional consultant.

The suggestions in this publication for recommended oils for ailments should never be in place of medical care and not all suggested oils will work for everyone.

Karen Ashton
THE ESSENTIAL OILS GUIDE

Essential Oils A – Z

Essential Oil Name

Basil

Image

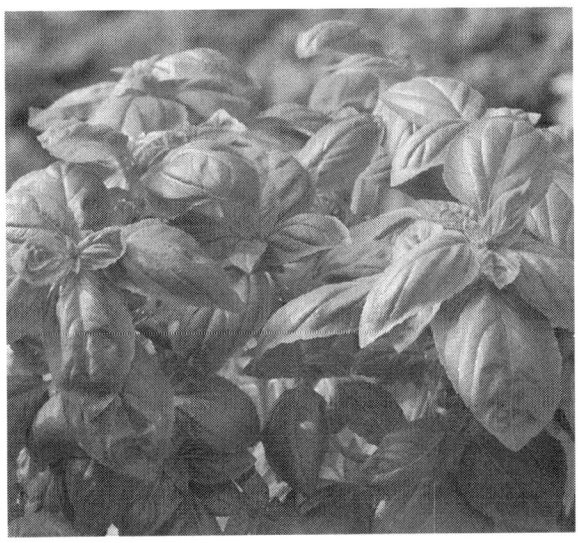

Botanical Name

Ocimum basilicum

Plant

Herb

Karen Ashton
THE ESSENTIAL OILS GUIDE

Plant Family

Lamiaceae (Labiatae)

Category

Herb

Note

Top

Objective

Uplift/Stimulation, Stress relief

Associated Planet

Mars

Extraction Method

Steam distillation

Main chemical constituents

Alcohols, Esters, Ketones, Oxides, Phenols, Monoterpenes, Sesquiterpenes

Karen Ashton
THE ESSENTIAL OILS GUIDE

Aroma

Clear, sweet, spicy, and herbaceous with a hint of aniseed

Properties

Analgesic, Antidepressant, Antiseptic, Antispasmodic, Antivenomous, Aphrodisiac, Bactericide, Carminative, Cephalic, Digestive, Emmenagogue, Expectorant, Febrifuge, Galactagogue, Insecticide, Nervine, Restorative, Stimulant, Stomachic, Sudorific, Tonic, Vermifuge

Contra-Indications / Precautions

- Can cause skin irritation, may be best to avoid using in a bath
- Not to be used during pregnancy

Benefits Body Systems

Circulatory system – hypotension, palpitations
Digestive system – antiseptic to the intestines, anti-spasmodic, colic, digestive problems, indigestion, nausea
Endocrine system – adrenal cortex stimulator
Muscular system – aches & pains, cramp, overworked muscles
Nervous system – epilepsy, nervous disorders

Karen Ashton
THE ESSENTIAL OILS GUIDE

Reproductive system – engorged painful breasts, scanty periods
Respiratory system – bronchitis, chest infections, fever, flu, head colds, sinusitis, whooping cough
Skeletal system - gout
The skin – acne, congestion, refreshing, sluggish, tonic

Other healing properties

Fatigue, fever, headaches, jaundice, migraines, overall tonic, wasp / insect bites, weakness

Psychological / Emotional benefits

Anxiety, cephalic (clears the mind), depression, exhaustion, (calms) hysteria, mental fatigue, (poor) memory, nervous debility, nervous insomnia, stress, Uplifting

Karen Ashton
THE ESSENTIAL OILS GUIDE

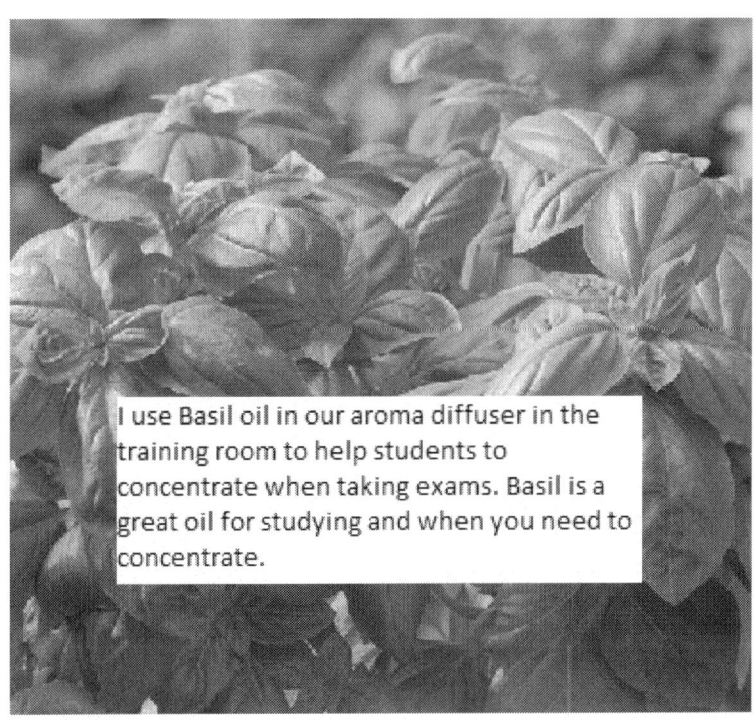

I use Basil oil in our aroma diffuser in the training room to help students to concentrate when taking exams. Basil is a great oil for studying and when you need to concentrate.

Karen Ashton
THE ESSENTIAL OILS GUIDE

Essential Oil Name

Benzoin

Image

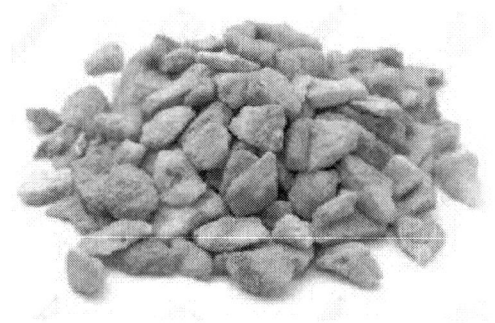

Botanical Name

Styrax benzoin

Plant

Balsam

Plant Family

Styracaceae

Category

Resin

Karen Ashton
THE ESSENTIAL OILS GUIDE

Note

Base

Objective

Relaxation, Stress relief

Associated Planet

Sun

Extraction Method

Solvent Extraction

Main chemical constituents

Acids, Aldehydes, Esters

Aroma

Sweet, Vanilla like

Properties

Antiseptic, Astringent, Carminative, Cephalic, Cordial, Deodorant, Diuretic, Expectorant, Sedative, Vulnerary

Karen Ashton
THE ESSENTIAL OILS GUIDE

Contra-Indications / Precautions

- Hypersensitive skin, diseased or damaged skin
- Has a drowsy effect, not suitable before driving or operating machinery

Benefits Body Systems

Circulatory system – warms the heart & circulation
Digestive system – blood sugar levels, colic, constipation, flatulence, heartburn, strengthens the pancreas, mouth ulcers
Endocrine system - diabetes
Lymphatic system – fluid retention
Muscular system – eases aches and pains,
Reproductive system – leucorrhoea, premature ejaculation,
Respiratory system – asthma, bronchitis, coughs & colds, flu, laryngitis, mucous problems, sore throats, tonic to the lungs,
Skeletal system – arthritis, rheumatism
The skin – athlete's foot, chapped skin, chilblains, cuts, dermatitis, dry skin, elasticity, healing, inflamed, irritated, mature, rashes, sores, wounds,
Urinary system – antiseptic, astringent, cystitis, diuretic, urinary tract infections, urine flow

Karen Ashton
THE ESSENTIAL OILS GUIDE

Other healing properties

Arthritis, rheumatism, sexual difficulties

Psychological / Emotional benefits

Anxiety, loneliness, nervous tension, stress, worry

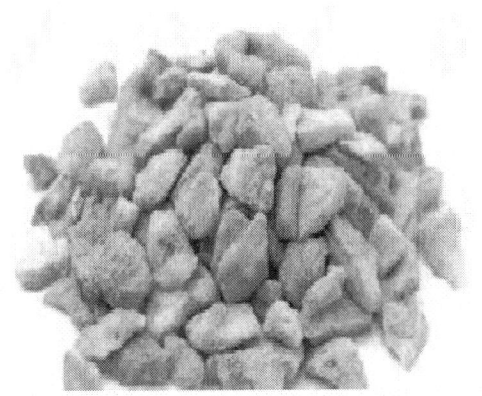

Benzoin is a resin & is thick in consistency so may not pass through the dropper top. I tend to remove the dropper top and use a pipette to count the correct number of drops into my blend.

Karen Ashton
THE ESSENTIAL OILS GUIDE

Essential Oil Name

Bergamot

Image

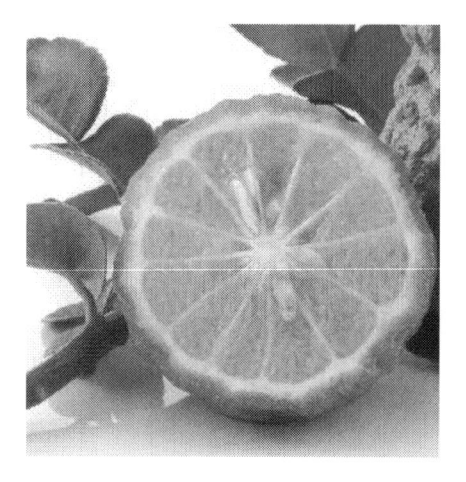

Botanical Name

Citrus bergamia Risso

Plant

Fruit

Plant Family

Ruttaceae

Karen Ashton
THE ESSENTIAL OILS GUIDE

Category

Citrus

Note

Top

Objective

Balancing, Stress relief

Associated Planet

No associated planets

Extraction Method

Cold expression

Main chemical constituents

Aliphatic aldehydes, Alcohols, Esters, Lactones, Monoterpenes, Sesquiterpenes

Aroma

Citrus with slight floral. light, refreshing.

Karen Ashton
THE ESSENTIAL OILS GUIDE

Properties

Analgesic, Antidepressant, Antiseptic, Antispasmodic, Carminative, Cicatrisant, Cordial, Deodorant, Digestive, Expectorant, Febrifuge, Insecticide, Sedative, Stomachic, Tonic, Vermifuge, Vulnerary.

Contra-Indications / Precautions

- Not suitable for epileptics
- Phototoxic, sunburn
- May not be suitable for hypersensitive skin

Benefits Body Systems

Circulatory system – stimulates circulation
Digestive system – regulates appetite, bile stimulant, colic, constipation, dyspepsia, eating disorders, flatulence, gall stones, gastric secretions, indigestion, intestinal parasites, spasms
Lymphatic system – fever
Muscular system – aches
Nervous system – calms the sympathetic nervous system, tonic
Reproductive system – candida, leucorrhoea, PMS, sexually transmitted diseases
Respiratory system – breathing difficulties, bronchitis, colds, flu, respiratory infections, tonsillitis, tuberculosis
The skin – acne, antiseptic, cold sores, chicken pox, eczema, healing, herpes, infections, infestations, itching,

oily skin, parasites, psoriasis, rashes, scabies, seborrhoea, shingles, sores, varicose ulcers, wounds, **Urinary system** – antiseptic, cystitis, inflammation, thrush, tonic effect, urinary tract infections

Other healing properties

Fever, insect repellent, keeps pets away from plants

Psychological / Emotional benefits

Agitation, anger, anxiety, balancing, claustrophobia, depression, eating disorders, frustration, grief, impatience, indecision, insecurity, insomnia, mood swings, negativity, sadness, sedative, stress, tantrum, (nervous) tension, uplifting

Karen Ashton
THE ESSENTIAL OILS GUIDE

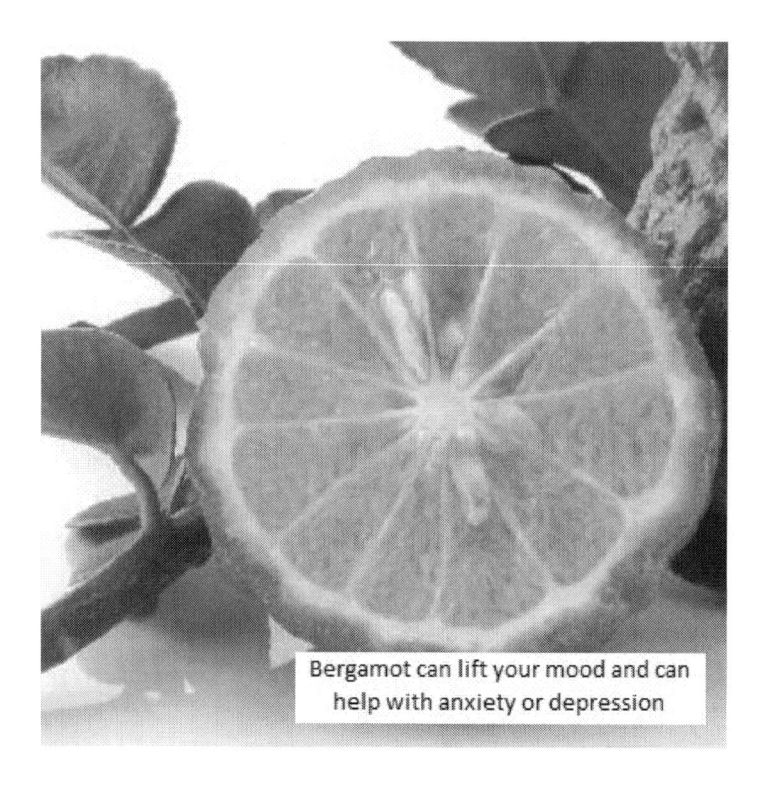

Bergamot can lift your mood and can help with anxiety or depression

Karen Ashton
THE ESSENTIAL OILS GUIDE

Essential Oil Name

Black Pepper

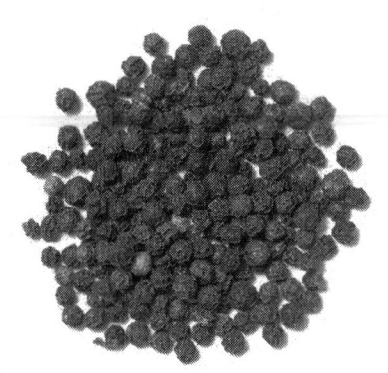

Image

Botanical Name

Piper nigrum

Plant

Fruit

Plant Family

Piperaceae

Category

Spice

Karen Ashton
THE ESSENTIAL OILS GUIDE

Note

Middle

Objective

Balancing

Associated Planet

Mars

Extraction Method

Distillation

Main chemical constituents

Aldehydes, Ketones, Oxides, Monoterpenes, Sesquiterpenes

Aroma

Spicy & Sharp, Warm

Properties

Analgesic, Antiemetic, Antiseptic, Antispasmodic, Aphrodisiac, Cardiac, Carminative, Detoxicant, Digestive, Diuretic, Febrifuge, Laxative, Rubefacient, Stimulant, Stomachic, Tonic

Karen Ashton
THE ESSENTIAL OILS GUIDE

Contra-Indications / Precautions

- May overstimulate the kidneys if used in excess
- May cause skin irritation

Benefits Body Systems

Circulatory system – anaemia, circulation, dilate blood vessels, new blood cells
Digestive system – appetite loss, bowel problems, colic, constipation, digestion of protein & fat, flatulence, heartburn, indigestion, nausea, peristalsis, saliva flow, spasms, stimulates the appetite, tonic to the stomach, vomiting, wind,
Lymphatic system – fluid retention
Muscular system – aches and pains, back ache, sprain, stiffness, tired & achy limbs,
Nervous system – sciatica, stimulant, vertigo
Reproductive system – period pains,
Respiratory system – catarrh, colds, flu, respiratory illnesses, sinusitis
Skeletal system – arthritis, rheumatism, tired & achy limbs, tone to skeletal muscles,
The skin – bruises, cellulite, perspiration, tone the skin
Urinary system – cystitis, diuretic, infections, stimulant to the kidneys, urine flow,

Karen Ashton
THE ESSENTIAL OILS GUIDE

Other healing properties

Fatigue, rheumatism, toothache, useful oil for sports after exertion, helps bring down temperature

Psychological / Emotional benefits

Aphrodisiac, balancing, exhaustion, mental fatigue, stamina, stimulant, strengthens & stimulates the mind, strengthens the nerves, warms the heart when you feel indifferent

Karen Ashton
THE ESSENTIAL OILS GUIDE

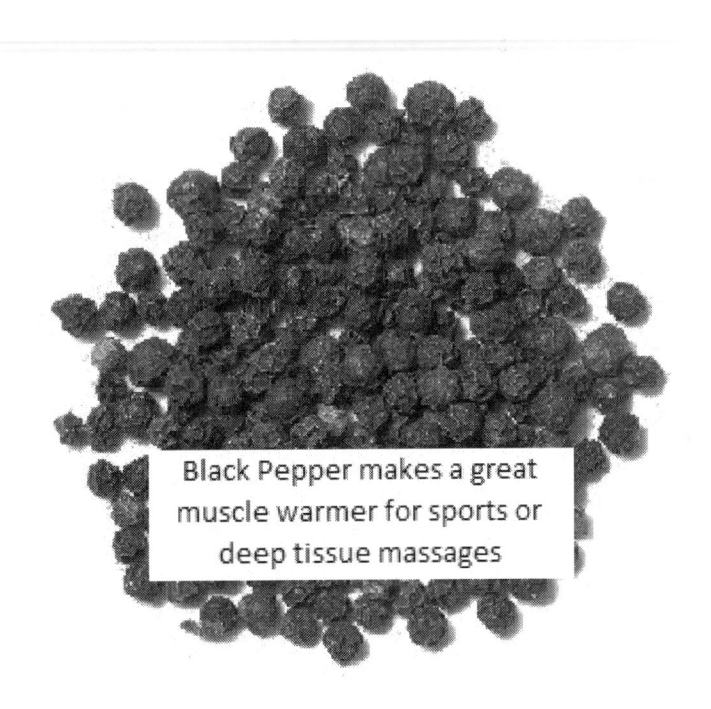

Black Pepper makes a great muscle warmer for sports or deep tissue massages

Karen Ashton
THE ESSENTIAL OILS GUIDE

Essential Oil Name

Cedarwood Atlas

Image

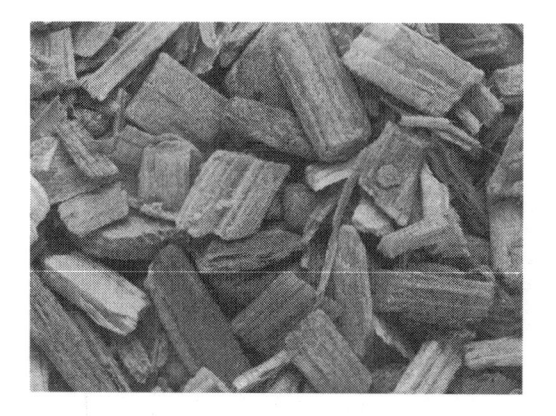

Botanical Name

Cedrus atlantica

Plant

Wood

Plant Family

Pinaceae

Karen Ashton
THE ESSENTIAL OILS GUIDE

Category

Tree

Note

Base

Objective

Balancing, Stress relief

Associated Planet

Sun

Extraction Method

Steam distillation

Main chemical constituents

Alcohols, Ketones, Sesquiterpenes

Aroma

Sweet, woody & musky

Karen Ashton
THE ESSENTIAL OILS GUIDE

Properties

Antiseptic, Astringent, Diuretic, Emollient, Expectorant, Fungicide, Insecticide, Sedative, Tonic

Contra-Indications / Precautions

- Could irritate the skin
- Best to avoid during pregnancy
- Do not use if undergoing chemotherapy

Benefits Body Systems

Circulatory system – pulmonary antiseptic, tonic to the circulation
Endocrine system – a tonic to the glandular system
Nervous system – a tonic to the nervous system
Reproductive system – leucorrhoea, PMT, regulates menstruation
Respiratory system – bronchitis, catarrh, coughs, expectorant, mucous
The skin – acne, alopecia, blemishes, dandruff, dermatitis, eczema, fungal infections, hair tonic, itching, oily skin, psoriasis, sebum balancer, spots, wounds/scabs/pus
Urinary system – antiseptic, cystitis, tonic effect to the kidneys, urinary tract infections

Other healing properties

Mildly astringent, tonic for entire body, helps with long term physical complaints, restores homeostasis by helping to put the body back into balance, has a 'drying' effect

Psychological / Emotional benefits

Anxiety, fear, impatience, indecision, jealousy, mood swings, nervous tension, panic, self-control, stress

"You can't buy happiness, but you can buy essential oils"

Karen Ashton
THE ESSENTIAL OILS GUIDE

Essential Oil Name

Chamomile German / Chamomile Roman

Image

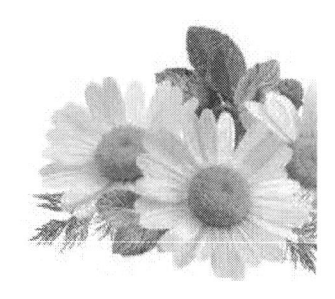

Botanical Name

Chamomile German - Matricaria recutita
Chamomile Roman – Anthemis nobilis

Plant

Flowers

Plant Family

Asteraceae (compositae)

Category

Flower

Karen Ashton
THE ESSENTIAL OILS GUIDE

Note

Middle

Objective

Relaxation, Stress relief

Associated Planet

Sun

Extraction Method

Steam distillation

Main chemical constituents

Alcohols, Esters, Oxides, Phenols, Monoterpenes, Sesquiterpenes

Aroma

Apple like

Properties

Analgesic, Anti-allergenic, Anticonvulsive, Antidepressant, Antiemetic, Antiphlogistic, Antipruritic, Antirheumatic, Antiseptic, Antispasmodic, Carminative, Cholagogue, Cicatrisant, Digestive, Diuretic, Emollient,

Karen Ashton
THE ESSENTIAL OILS GUIDE

Emmenagogue, Febrifuge, Hepatic, Nervine, Sedative, Splenetic, Stomachic, Sudorific, Tonic, Vermifuge, Vulnerary

Contra-Indications / Precautions

- Best avoided during early stages of pregnancy due to its emmenagogue properties
- Could cause dermatitis

Benefits Body Systems

Circulatory system – anaemia, blood vessel constriction, thread veins
Digestive system – appetite loss, bile stimulation, colic, colitis, diarrhoea, gastritis, haemorrhoids, heartburn, IBS, inflammation of the bowels, nausea, intestinal parasites, liver congestion, peptic ulcer, upset stomach, spasms, vomiting
Lymphatic system – fluid retention, leucocyte production, spleen congestion
Muscular system – aches, back ache, muscle pain, spasms, sprains, strengthens the tissue
Nervous system – earache, headache, migraine, neuralgia, sedating, sciatica, toothache,
Reproductive system – menstrual pain, period pain, PMS, menopausal
Respiratory system – asthma, cough (tickly), hay fever
Skeletal – arthritis, inflamed joints, rheumatism, sprains

Karen Ashton
THE ESSENTIAL OILS GUIDE

The skin – acne, allergic skin, bacteria, blisters, boils, bruises, burns, cracked nipples, chicken pox itching, cleansing, dermatitis, dry skin, eczema, elasticity, eye infections, flaky skin, healing, herpes, hives, hypersensitive skin, inflammation, itchiness, jaundice, nappy rash, perspiration (induce), psoriasis, puffiness, sensitive skin, scalp tonic, thread veins, ulcers, wounds
Urinary system – cystitis, urinary tract disorders

Other healing properties

Boosts immune system, fights bacteria, headaches, Infections, Inflammation, Insect bites, Insomnia, tonic, white blood cell production

Psychological / Emotional benefits

Anger, agitation, anxiety, calms the mind, depression, fear, frustration, hysteria, insomnia, irritability, nervous complaints, panic, patience, peace, relaxant, shock, stress, tantrum, tension, (allays) worries

"I have enough essential oils, said no one ever!"

Essential Oil Name

Clary Sage

Image

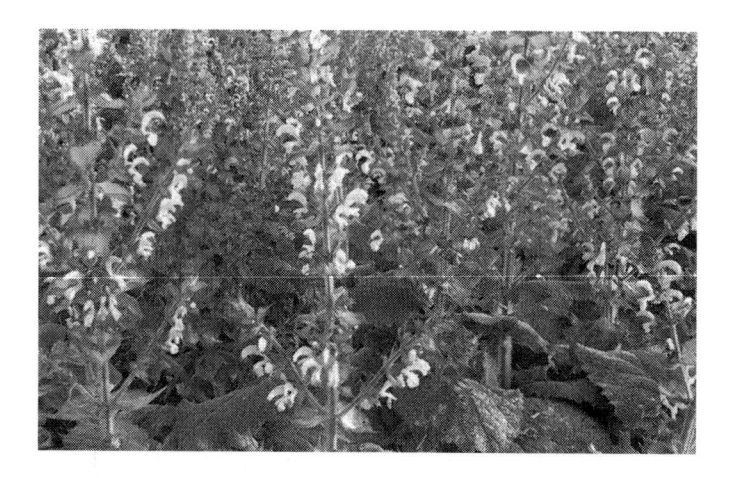

Botanical Name

Salvia sclarea

Plant

Herb

Plant Family

Lamiaceae (Labiatae)

Karen Ashton
THE ESSENTIAL OILS GUIDE

Category

Herb

Note

Middle

Objective

Balancing, Stress relief

Associated Planet

Moon / Mercury

Extraction Method

Steam distillation

Main chemical constituents

Alcohol, Ester, Oxides, Monoterpenes, Sesquiterpenes

Aroma

Strong, herbal / nutty

Karen Ashton
THE ESSENTIAL OILS GUIDE

Properties

Anticonvulsive, Antidepressant, Antiphlogistic, Antiseptic, Antispasmodic, Antisudorific, Aphrodisiac, Balsamic, Carminative, Deodorant, Digestive, Emmenagogue, Hypotensive, Nervine, Parturient, Sedative, Stomachic, Tonic, Uterine

Contra-Indications / Precautions

- **Antisudorific** Do not use before driving or operating machinery as extremely sedative
- Could cause headaches if used excessively
- May cause nausea
- Do not use during pregnancy
- Avoid alcohol as can induce nausea

Benefits Body Systems

Circulatory system – hypertension, varicose veins, vasoconstrictor
Digestive system – calming, colic, cramps, flatulence, gastric spasms, indigestion, soothing, wind
Endocrine system – hormone balancing
Muscular system – muscle relaxant, spasms, cramps, tension
Nervous system – epilepsy, headaches, migraines
Reproductive system – dysmenorrhoea, fertility problems through stress, hot flushes, irregular periods,

Karen Ashton
THE ESSENTIAL OILS GUIDE

can help during labour, menopause, period pains, PMT, sexual problems, tonic for the womb, uterus problems
Respiratory system – asthma, coughs, sore throats
The skin – acne, bacteria, cell regeneration, dandruff, greasy hair, hair growth, healing, inflammation, odour (deodorant), oily skin, excessive perspiration, puffiness, sebum production (controls), scalp problems, scalp tonic
Urinary system – tonic to the kidneys

Other healing properties

Boosting for the immune system, convalescence, dreaming (may heighten), drowsy, headaches, sedative

Psychological / Emotional benefits

Anxiety, balancing, claustrophobia, (brings about a) euphoric state, grief, hysteria, insomnia, irritation, loneliness, mood swings, negativity, nervous tension, panicky states, helps to see things in perspective, (can help with) post-natal depression, racing mind, relaxant, restlessness, sedative, stress, tantrum, uplifting, worry

"I don't need an inspirational quote! I need essential oils"

Karen Ashton
THE ESSENTIAL OILS GUIDE

Essential Oil Name

Cypress

Image

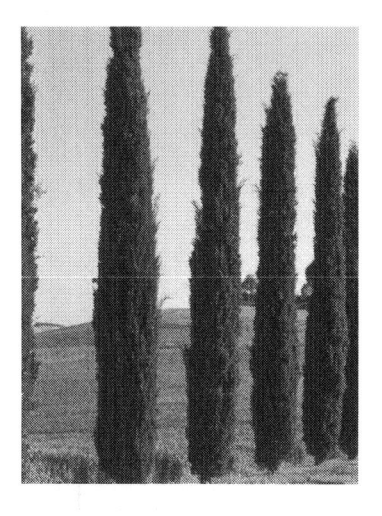

Botanical Name

Cupressus Sempervirens

Plant

Twigs

Plant Family

Cupressaceae

Karen Ashton
THE ESSENTIAL OILS GUIDE

Category

Tree

Note

Middle

Objective

Relaxation, Stress relief

Associated Planet

Saturn

Extraction Method

Steam distillation

Main chemical constituents

Alcohols, Esters, Oxides, Monoterpenes, Sesquiterpenes

Aroma

Woody, spicy & refreshing

Karen Ashton
THE ESSENTIAL OILS GUIDE

Properties

Antirheumatic, Antiseptic, Antispasmodic, Antisudorific, Astringent, Cicatrisant, Deodorant, Diuretic, Febrifuge, Haemostatic, Hepatic, Insecticide, Restorative, Sedative, Styptic, Tonic, Vasoconstrictor

Contra-Indications / Precautions

- Best avoided during pregnancy as regulates blood flow
- May not be suitable for people with high blood pressure

Benefits Body Systems

Circulatory system – regulates blood flow, thread veins, a tonic to the circulatory system, varicose veins, vasoconstriction
Digestive system – haemorrhoids, a tonic to the liver
Endocrine system – hormonal imbalances
Lymphatic system – diuretic, fluid retention, oedema
Muscular system – muscle cramps
Nervous system – balancing to the nerves
Reproductive system – heavy menstruation / menstrual problems, menopausal problems, ovaries (regulates)
Respiratory system – asthma, bronchitis, coughs, flu, whooping cough
Skeletal system – rheumatism

Karen Ashton
THE ESSENTIAL OILS GUIDE

The skin – balancing, cellulite, dehydrated skin, mature skin, oily skin, perspiration (excessive), warts, watery, wound healing
Urinary system – diuretic, incontinence

Other healing properties

Rheumatism

Psychological / Emotional benefits

(Soothes) anger, bereavement, calming, fear, grief, guilt, irritability, jealousy, (helps to remove) nervous tension, psychic blocks, sadness, stress

"The best time for new beginnings is now"

Karen Ashton
THE ESSENTIAL OILS GUIDE

Essential Oil Name

Eucalyptus

Image

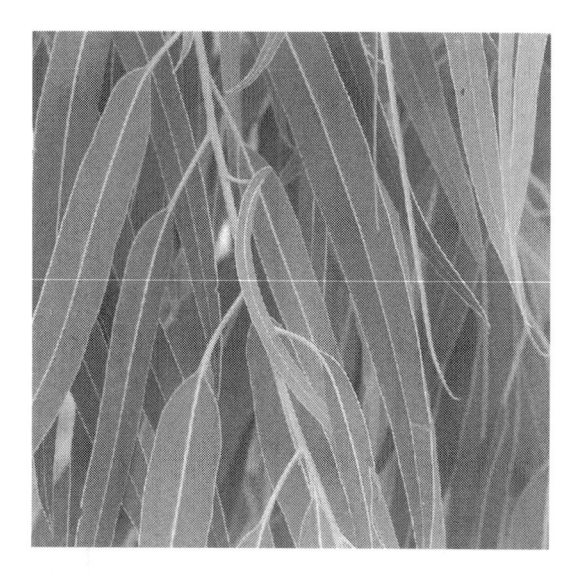

Botanical Name

Eucalyptus globulus

Plant

Leaves

Karen Ashton
THE ESSENTIAL OILS GUIDE

Plant Family

Myrtaceae

Category

Tree

Note

Top

Objective

Uplift/Stimulation

Associated Planet

No associated

Extraction Method

Steam distillation

Main chemical constituents

Aldehyde, Alcohols, Ketones, Oxides, Monoterpenes

Aroma

Sharp & piercing

Karen Ashton
THE ESSENTIAL OILS GUIDE

Properties

Analgesic, Antirheumatic, Antiphlogistic, Antiseptic, Antispasmodic, Antiviral, Bactericide, Balsamic, Cicatrisant, Decongestant, Deodorant, Depurative, Diuretic, Expectorant, Febrifuge, Hypoglycaemia, Insecticide, Rubefacient, Stimulant, Vermifuge, Vulnerary

Contra-Indications / Precautions

- Care should be taken to not overuse as a powerful oil
- Best avoided if high blood pressure
- Do not use if have epilepsy
- This oil may antidote homeopathic remedies

Benefits Body Systems

Circulatory system – circulation, hypotension
Digestive system – Diarrhoea
Endocrine system – Diabetes (stimulates the pancreas)
Lymphatic system - fevers
Muscular system – muscular aches, pains, sprain
Nervous system – headaches, migraine, neuralgia, sciatica, strengthening
Reproductive system – candida
Respiratory system – antiviral, asthma, bronchitis, catarrh, chest infection, colds, coughs, flu, hay fever,

inflammation, mucus, sinusitis, throat infections, tuberculosis
Skeletal system – Rheumatism
The skin – athlete's foot, burns, congestion, healing, infections, lice, scarring, spots, toxins, wounds
Urinary system – antiseptic, cystitis,

Other healing properties

Anti-viral, fever, headaches, insect bites, insect repellent, helps to prevent disease, rheumatism

Psychological / Emotional benefits

Clears the head, cooling on the emotions, helps with concentration

Karen Ashton
THE ESSENTIAL OILS GUIDE

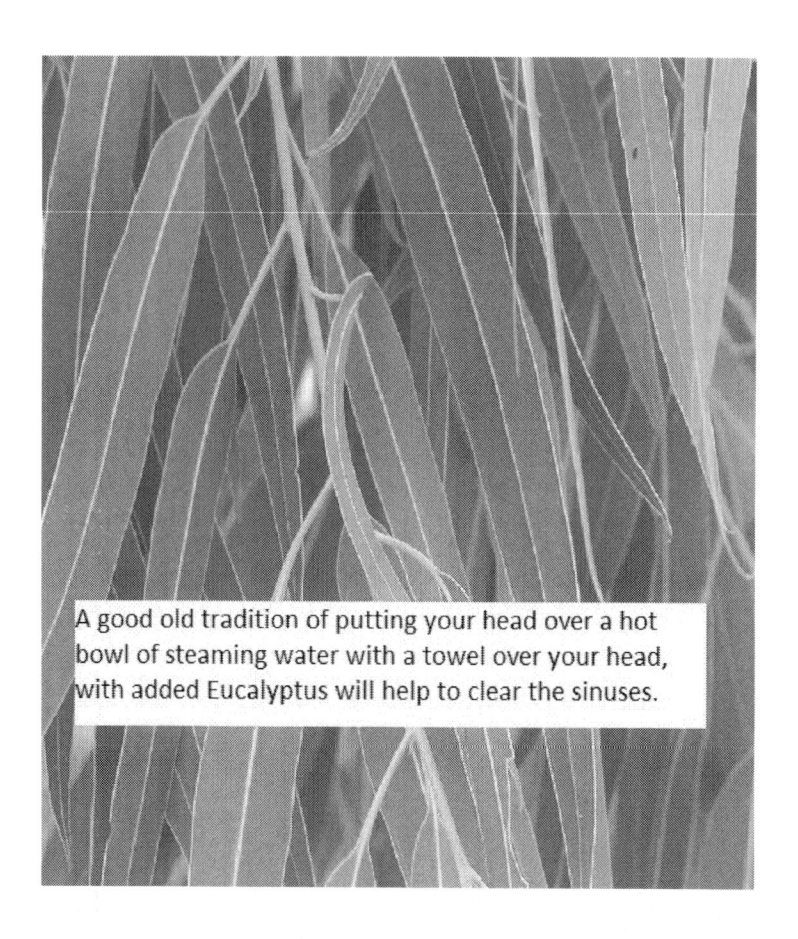

A good old tradition of putting your head over a hot bowl of steaming water with a towel over your head, with added Eucalyptus will help to clear the sinuses.

Karen Ashton
THE ESSENTIAL OILS GUIDE

Essential Oil Name

Fennel

Image

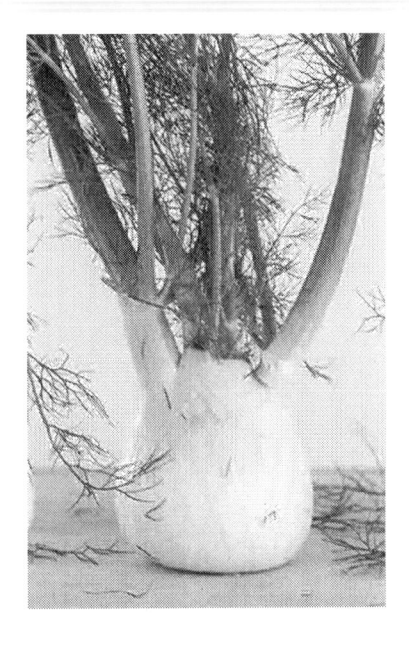

Botanical Name

Foeniculum vulgare

Plant

Fruit

Karen Ashton
THE ESSENTIAL OILS GUIDE

Plant Family

Apiaceae (umbellifera)

Category

Herb

Note

Middle

Objective

Uplift/Stimulation

Associated Planet

Mercury

Extraction Method

Steam distillation

Main chemical constituents

Acids, Alcohols, Aldehydes, Ketones, Oxides, Phenols, Monoterpenes

Karen Ashton
THE ESSENTIAL OILS GUIDE

Aroma

Herbal & Floral, slightly aniseed

Properties

Anti-microbial, Antiphlogistic, Antiseptic, Antispasmodic, Aperitif, Carminative, Detoxicant, Diuretic, Emmenagogue, Expectorant, Galactagogue, Insecticide, Laxative, Resolvent, Splenetic, Stimulant, Stomachic, Sudorific, Tonic, Vermifuge

Contra-Indications / Precautions

- Do not over-use as could be toxic
- Hypersensitive skin
- Epilepsy
- Pregnancy
- Children
- Do not use if undergoing chemotherapy

Benefits Body Systems

Circulatory system – circulation, combats blood / organ impurities
Digestive system – colic, constipation, dyspepsia, eating disorders, flatulence, hiccups, indigestion, nausea, tonic to the liver & digestive system, vomiting
Endocrine system – activate the glandular system
Lymphatic system – cellulitis, fluid retention, oedema

Karen Ashton
THE ESSENTIAL OILS GUIDE

Muscular system – muscle tone
Nervous system – Calming on the nervous system
Reproductive system – Amenorrhoea, hormone oestrogen, irregular periods, menopausal problems, menstruation, low sex drive, PMT
Respiratory system – Asthma, bronchitis, cold, coughs, hiccups, whooping cough
Skeletal system – Joints, rheumatism
The skin – bruises, cellulite, cleansing, congested skin, elasticity, mature skin, muscle tone, oily skin, tonic, wrinkles
Urinary system – kidney stones, tonic to the kidneys

Other healing properties

Body cleanser, helps to rid the body of food & alcohol toxins, hangovers, a tonic to the spleen, insect bites, a diuretic, can help with nursing mothers, obesity, rheumatism

Psychological / Emotional benefits

Courage, longevity, strength

Karen Ashton
THE ESSENTIAL OILS GUIDE

Essential Oil Name

Frankincense

Image

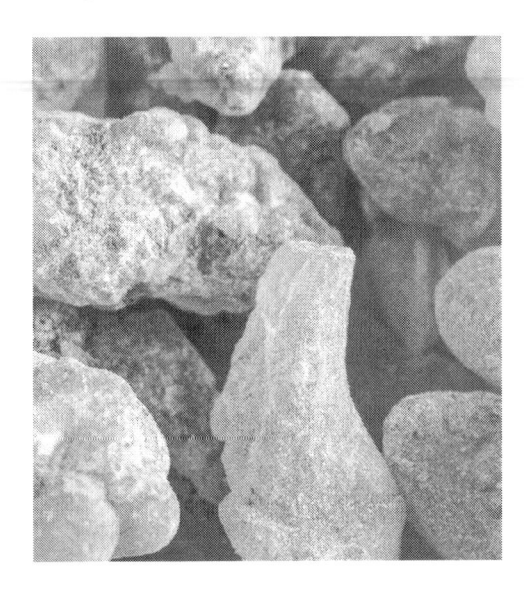

Botanical Name

Boswellia sacra

Plant

Resin

Karen Ashton
THE ESSENTIAL OILS GUIDE

Plant Family

Burseraceae

Category

Resin

Note

Base

Objective

Relaxation, Stress relief

Associated Planet

Sun

Extraction Method

Steam distillation

Main chemical constituents

Alcohol, Esters, Monoterpenes, Sesquiterpenes

Aroma

Warm, woody & spicy

Karen Ashton
THE ESSENTIAL OILS GUIDE

Properties

Anti-inflammatory, Antiseptic, Astringent, Carminative, Cicatrisant, Cytophalactic, Digestive, Diuretic, Sedative, Tonic, Uterine, Vulnerary

Contra-Indications / Precautions

- No precautions as such

Benefits Body Systems

Digestive system – belching, dyspepsia, indigestion, soothing
Reproductive system – Amenorrhoea, dysmenorrhoea, genital infections, labour, leucorrhoea, PMS, tonic to the uterus
Respiratory system – asthma, breathing (slows it down), breathlessness, bronchitis, catarrh, colds, coughs (palliative), flu, laryngitis, lung (helps to clear), mucous
The skin – ageing skin, astringent, balancing, combination skin, dermatitis, eczema, inflammation, mature skin, oily skin, psoriasis, rejuvenating, scar tissue, slack skin, sores, sunburn, tonic to the skin, ulcers, wounds, wrinkles
Urinary system – cystitis, tonic

Karen Ashton
THE ESSENTIAL OILS GUIDE

Psychological / Emotional benefits

Anger, anxiety, bereavement, calming to the emotions, claustrophobia, comforting, fear, frustration, hysteria, impatience, insomnia, nervous tension, obsessions of the past, panic, (could help with) postnatal depression, refreshing, restlessness, shock, soothes and elevates the mind, stress, worry

Karen Ashton
THE ESSENTIAL OILS GUIDE

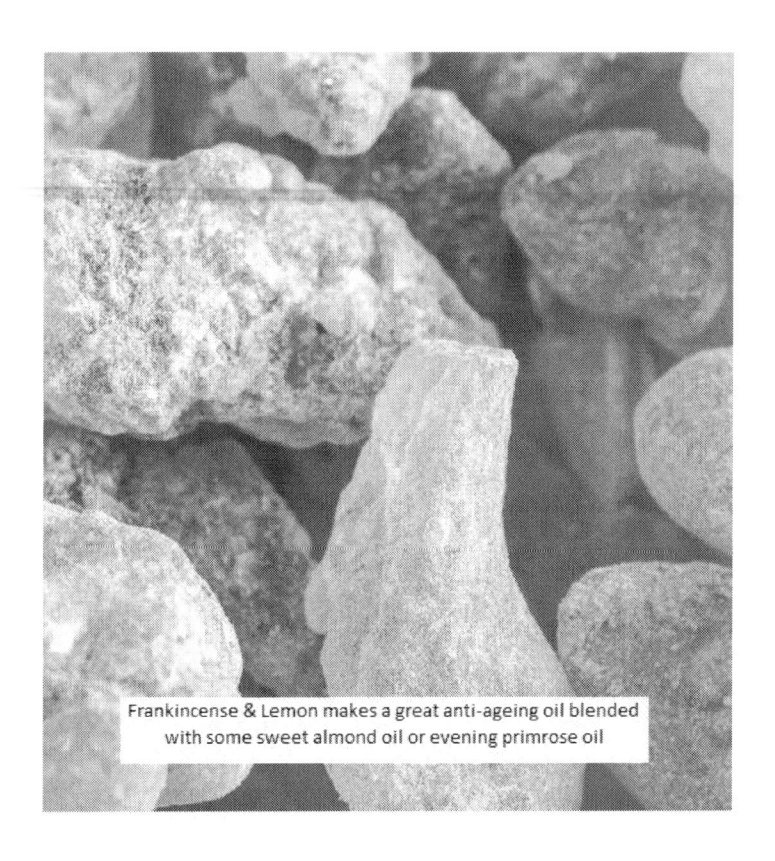

Frankincense & Lemon makes a great anti-ageing oil blended with some sweet almond oil or evening primrose oil

Karen Ashton
THE ESSENTIAL OILS GUIDE

Essential Oil Name

Geranium

Image

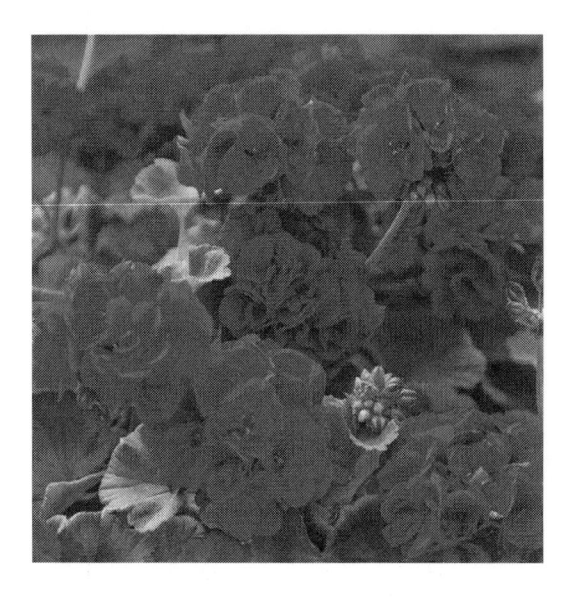

Botanical Name

Pelargonium Graveolens

Plant

Leaves

Karen Ashton
THE ESSENTIAL OILS GUIDE

Plant Family

Geraniaceae

Category

Flower

Note

Middle

Objective

Balancing, Stress relief

Associated Planet

Venus

Extraction Method

Steam distillation

Main chemical constituents

Aldehydes, Alcohols, Esters, Ketones, Oxides, Monoterpenes, Sesquiterpenes

Karen Ashton
THE ESSENTIAL OILS GUIDE

Aroma

Sweet, but heavy. Rose-like

Properties

Analgesic, Anticoagulant, Antidepressant, Antiseptic, Astringent, Cicatrisant, Cytophalactic, Diuretic, Deodorant, Haemostatic, Hypoglycaemia, Insecticide, Styptic, Tonic, Vasoconstrictor, Vulnerary

Contra-Indications / Precautions

- Hypersensitive skin / dermatitis
- Pregnancy
- Could cause restlessness if used in excess

Benefits Body Systems

Circulatory system – bleeding (slows), blood flow, circulation, thread veins, varicose veins
Digestive system – balancing, colitis, diarrhoea, gallstones, gastric problems, gastritis, stimulant / tonic to the gall bladder & liver, ulcers
Endocrine system – Adrenal cortex balancer, diabetes, hormones (regulates)
Lymphatic system – cellulitis, fluid retention, oedema, stimulates the lymphatic system, toxins & waste

Karen Ashton
THE ESSENTIAL OILS GUIDE

Nervous system – neuralgia
Reproductive system – menopausal problems, heavy periods, PMT, secretion, tonic
Respiratory system – infections, mouth infections, mucous, throat
The skin – antiseptic, astringent, athletes' foot, balancing, burns, cellulite, chilblains, cleanser, cold sores, combination skin, congestion, eczema, head lice, herpes, jaundice, oily skin, scar tissue, sebum balancing, shingles, sluggishness, sunburn, tonic, wounds
Urinary system – cystitis, diuretic, kidney stones, tonic to the kidneys, urinary infections

Other healing properties

Addictive states, inflammation, insect repellent, jet lag, pain relief

Psychological / Emotional benefits

Anger, claustrophobia, depression, insecurity, irritability, mood swings/ balancing, nervous tension, stress, uplifting

Karen Ashton
THE ESSENTIAL OILS GUIDE

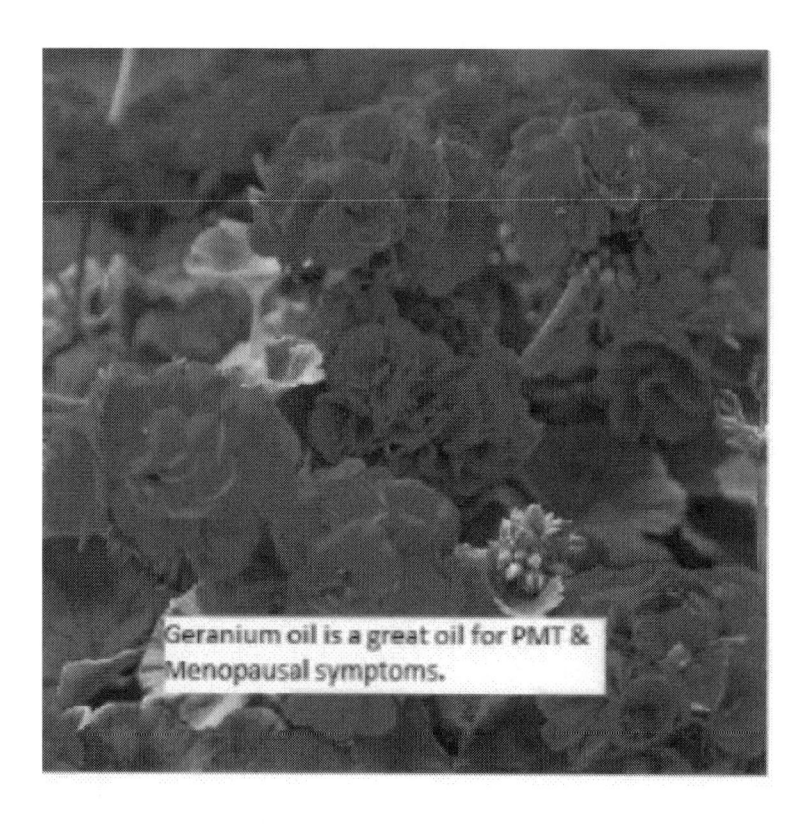

Geranium oil is a great oil for PMT & Menopausal symptoms.

Karen Ashton
THE ESSENTIAL OILS GUIDE

Essential Oil Name

Ginger

Image

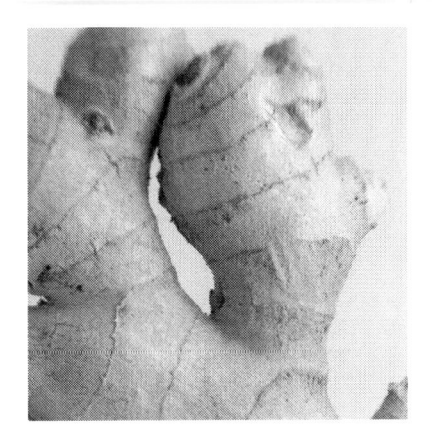

Botanical Name

Zingiber officinale

Plant

Rhizome

Plant Family

Zingiberaceae

Category

Spice

Note

Base

Objective

Uplift/Stimulation

Associated Planet

Mars

Extraction Method

Steam distillation

Main chemical constituents

Alcohols, Aldehydes, Ketones, Oxides, Monoterpenes, Sesquiterpenes

Aroma

Spicy, Sweet, Warm

Karen Ashton
THE ESSENTIAL OILS GUIDE

Properties

Analgesic, Antiemetic, Antiseptic, Antiscorbutic, Aperitif, Aphrodisiac, Bactericide, Carminative, Expectorant, Febrifuge, Laxative, Rubefacient, Stimulant, Stomachic, Sudorific, Tonic

Contra-Indications / Precautions

- Hypersensitive skin

Benefits Body Systems

Circulatory system – angina, cholesterol, circulation, clotting, fever, tonic to the heart, tonic to the blood and varicose veins
Digestive system – appetite loss, colic, diarrhoea, flatulence, gastric juice flow, indigestion, nausea, settling & toning, sickness (incl., travel)
Muscular system – aches, cramp, muscle spasms, pains
Reproductive system – aphrodisiac, impotence, period regulator
Respiratory system – catarrh, colds (runny), coughs, fever, flu, shivers, sinusitis, sore throats, tonsillitis
Skeletal system – arthritis, rheumatism
The skin – bruises, increases sweating, sweat glands

Other healing properties

Hangovers, jet lag, rheumatism, sharpens the senses, warming action so good with damp conditions

Psychological / Emotional benefits

Cheering, grounding, indecision, (Can help with) memory, mental fatigue, nervous exhaustion, self-control, sharpens the senses, stimulating, tiredness, warming to the emotions

Karen Ashton
THE ESSENTIAL OILS GUIDE

Ginger & Lemon for joint pain

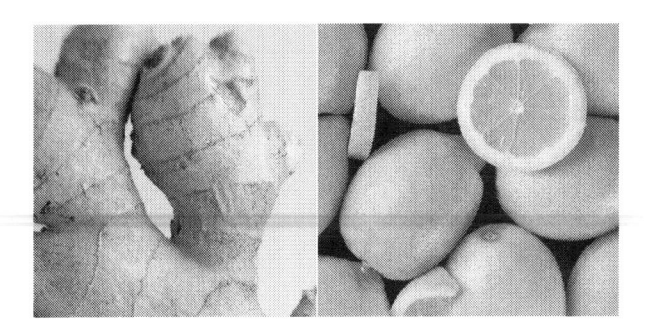

I had suffered from hip joint pain for 4 years, and after many appointments with doctors, consultants and physiotherapists, I was finally diagnosed with severe osteoarthritis and ulcerated bone in my right hip. Autumn of 2018, I was finally referred to Exeter hospital for a hip replacement, after being turned down by doctors on several occasions. The wait for surgery was 12 months, so my husband self-referred me to The Plymouth Trust, what an amazing service! He self-referred me in December, I attended a pre-op appointment at the end of January, and my operation took place on March 22nd, 2019! Amazing service and I am now in my 3rd week of recovery and doing well.

But, what did I do to get me through the joint pain before the op? Ginger and Lemon was my answer! I stayed away from pain killer medication as much as I could and 'went cold turkey', but to help me through this I would make up a blend of ginger and lemon essential oils with either grapeseed or sweet almond oil

Karen Ashton
THE ESSENTIAL OILS GUIDE

and I would massage it onto my hip. Ginger is a great anti-inflammatory oil and good for muscular and joint pain. Lemon oil is a great detoxifying oil and helped to take those toxins away from the area. Lemon oil is also an uplifting & cooling oil so in those times when the pain and restriction of movement got me down, the Lemon oil would give me a boost. Ginger oil is also warming to the emotions and helped in times when I felt down.

Instead of using essential oils, I sometimes used fresh ginger, crushed into a pulp and mixed with fresh lemon juice. The pulp mixture was then applied to my hip and I drank the rest, so it would take affect internally and externally.

Karen Ashton
THE ESSENTIAL OILS GUIDE

Essential Oil Name

Grapefruit

Image

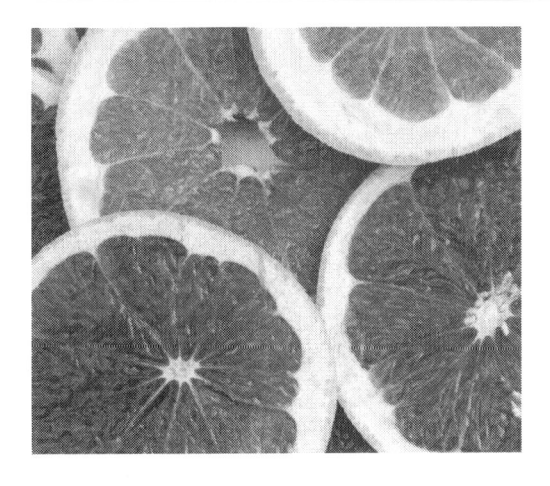

Botanical Name

Citrus Paradisi

Plant

Fruit

Plant Family

Ruttaceae

Karen Ashton
THE ESSENTIAL OILS GUIDE

Category

Citrus

Note

Top

Objective

Uplift/Stimulation, Stress relief

Associated Planet

Sun

Extraction Method

Cold expression

Main chemical constituents

Alcohol, Aldehyde, Esters, Lactones & coumarins, Monoterpenes, Sesquiterpenes

Aroma

Sharp, refreshing, tangy

Karen Ashton
THE ESSENTIAL OILS GUIDE

Properties

Antidepressant, Antiseptic, Aperitif, Diuretic, Disinfectant, Resolvent, Stimulant, Tonic

Contra-Indications / Precautions

- Could cause skin irritation in sunlight as photo-sensitive

Benefits Body Systems

Circulatory system – cleansing to the vascular system, nourishing to cells, toxins
Digestive system – Appetite stimulant, bile secretion, gall stones, liver tonic, obesity, tonic to the digestive system
Lymphatic system – detoxifying, diuretic, fluid retention, stimulant, toxins, water retention
Nervous system – balancing on the central nervous system, headaches, migraine
Reproductive system – PMT, pregnancy comforting
The skin – acne, cellulite, congestion, oily skin
Urinary system – cleansing & tonic to the kidneys

Karen Ashton
THE ESSENTIAL OILS GUIDE

Other healing properties

Antiseptic, cleansing, 'dissolving' properties, ear infections, headache, jet lag, soothing

Psychological / Emotional benefits

Anger, balancing to the emotions, confidence, depression, euphoric, hypnotic, indecision, manic-depression, nervous exhaustion, frustration, regret, reviving, sadness, stress, tiredness, uplifting

Karen Ashton
THE ESSENTIAL OILS GUIDE

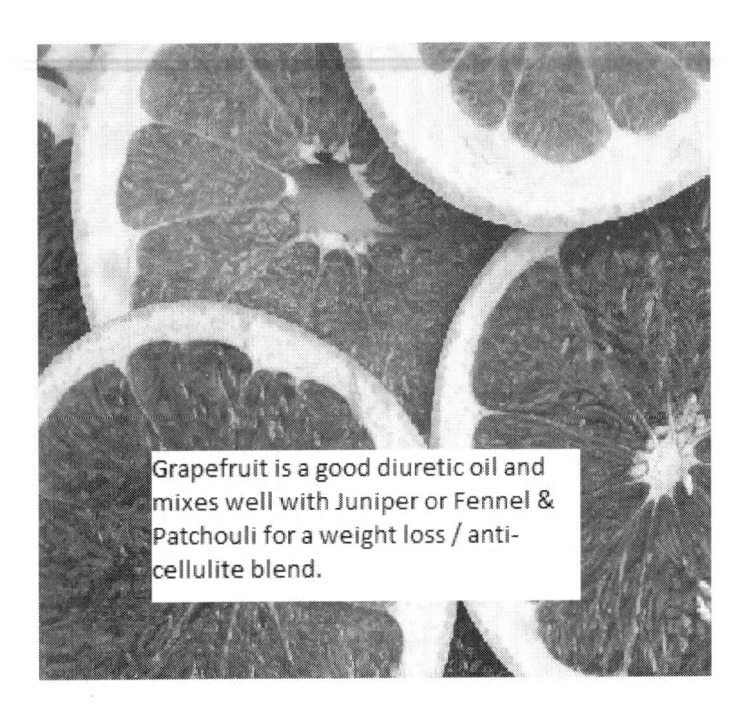

Grapefruit is a good diuretic oil and mixes well with Juniper or Fennel & Patchouli for a weight loss / anti-cellulite blend.

Karen Ashton
THE ESSENTIAL OILS GUIDE

Essential Oil Name

Jasmine

Image

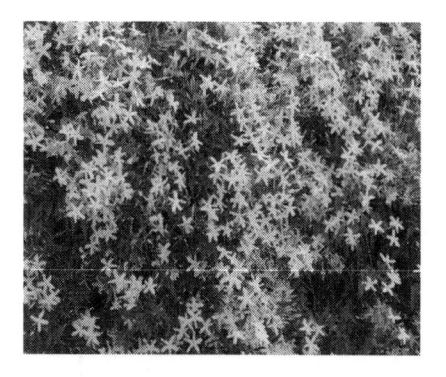

Botanical Name

Jasminum grandiflorum

Plant

Flowers

Plant Family

Oleaceae

Category

Flower

Karen Ashton
THE ESSENTIAL OILS GUIDE

Note

Base

Objective

Relaxation, Stress relief

Associated Planet

Jupiter

Extraction Method

Solvent extraction

Main chemical constituents

Alcohols, Esters, Indole, Ketones, Phenols

Aroma

Rich, sweet, floral & exotic

Properties

Antidepressant, Antiseptic, Antispasmodic, Aphrodisiac, Emollient, Galactagogue, Parturient, Sedative, Uterine

Karen Ashton
THE ESSENTIAL OILS GUIDE

Contra-Indications / Precautions

- Pregnancy (apart from labour)
- Overuse can disrupt bodily fluids
- Can affect concentration due to its relaxing properties
- Use in moderation as a powerful oil

Benefits Body Systems

Reproductive system – childbirth (can help with delivery), contractions (can strengthen but ease pain), fertility (can help to boost), frigidity, genital infections, impotence, labour pains, PMT, post-natal depression, tonic to the male reproductive system, uterine spasms, uterine tonic
Respiratory system – breathing (helps to deepen), catarrh, coughs (calming to irritant), hoarseness, laryngitis, spasms, upper respiratory tract infection
Skeletal system – stiff limbs
The skin – combination skin, dry skin, elasticity, irritated skin, scarring, sensitive skin, warming to the skin

Psychological / Emotional benefits

Bereavement, calms the nerves, confidence, depression, (restores) energy, euphoria, guilt, insecurity, (helps the feeling of) positivity, revitalising, self-control, stress, warms the emotions

Karen Ashton
THE ESSENTIAL OILS GUIDE

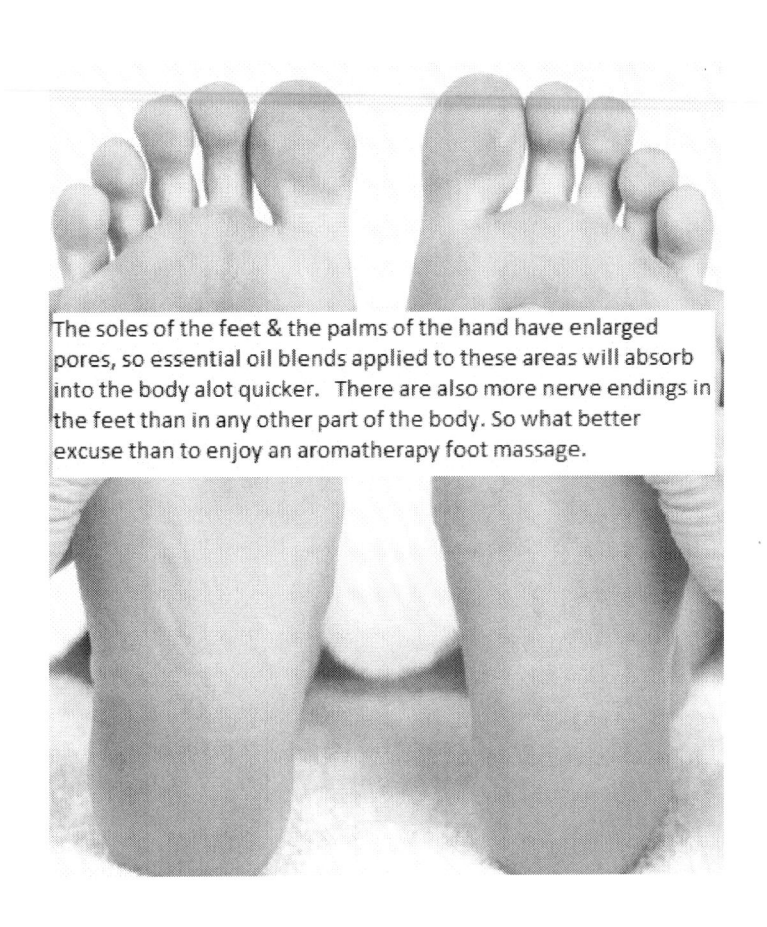

The soles of the feet & the palms of the hand have enlarged pores, so essential oil blends applied to these areas will absorb into the body alot quicker. There are also more nerve endings in the feet than in any other part of the body. So what better excuse than to enjoy an aromatherapy foot massage.

Karen Ashton
THE ESSENTIAL OILS GUIDE

Essential Oil Name

Juniper

Image

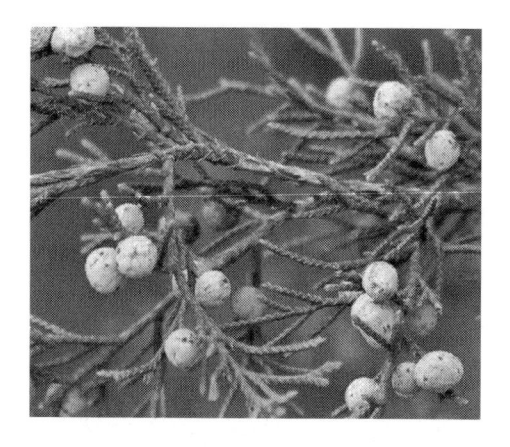

Botanical Name

Juniperus communis

Plant

Berry

Plant Family

Cupressaceae

Karen Ashton
THE ESSENTIAL OILS GUIDE

Category

Tree

Note

Middle

Objective

Balancing

Associated Planet

Sun

Extraction Method

Steam distillation

Main chemical constituents

Alcohol, Esters, Monoterpenes, Sesquiterpenes

Aroma

Refreshing & slightly woody/pine like, warm

Karen Ashton
THE ESSENTIAL OILS GUIDE

Properties

Antiseptic, Antirheumatic, Antispasmodic, Aphrodisiac, Astringent, Carminative, Cicatrisant, Depurative, Detoxicant, Disinfectant, Diuretic, Emmenagogue, Nervine, Insecticide, Parturient, Rubefacient, Stimulant, Stomachic, Sudorific, Tonic, Vulnerary

Contra-Indications / Precautions

- Prolonged use may overstimulate the kidneys
- Pregnancy

Benefits Body Systems

Circulatory system – circulation, purify the blood, stimulates the superficial circulation, varicose veins
Digestive system – appetite regulator / loss, colic, diarrhoea, tonic to the liver, toxins
Endocrine system - diabetes
Lymphatic system – cellulitis, detoxifying, diuretic, fluid retention, oedema, tonic to the spleen
Muscular system – aches & pains
Nervous system – calming, epilepsy, sciatica
Reproductive system – antiseptic for the genito-urinary tract, dysmenorrhoea, labour, menstrual cramps & cycle
Respiratory system – mucous

Karen Ashton
THE ESSENTIAL OILS GUIDE

Skeletal system – arthritis, gout, pain relief, rheumatism, sciatica, stiffness of joints
The skin – acne, blocked pores, congested skin tonic, dermatitis, diseases & disorders (Skin), eczema, infestations, oily skin & hair tonic, perspiration (increases), psoriasis, scar tissue, skin tone, wounds
Urinary system – antiseptic for the genito-urinary tract, cystitis, kidney stones / tonic, uric acid

Other healing properties

Can help with obesity, cellulite, rheumatism, stimulant when feeling drowsy, toxic build up (counter-effect), uric acid

Psychological / Emotional benefits

Anxiety, clearing, fear, guilt, insecurity, insomnia, loneliness, negativity, nervous stress & tension, sadness, strengthens the nerves, stress, supports the spirit when in challenging situations, worry

> **TIP:**
> What oils do you love or hate? What can you embrace or what are you avoiding? Have a look at the properties of these oils to give you an idea of what you are embracing or blocking!

Karen Ashton
THE ESSENTIAL OILS GUIDE

Essential Oil Name

Lavandin

Image

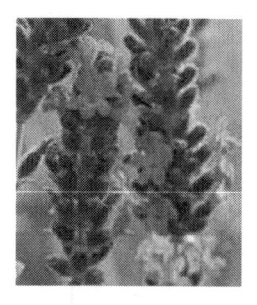

Botanical Name

Lavandula x intermedia Emeric ex Loisel

Plant

Flowers

Plant Family

Lamiaceae (Labiatae)

Category

Flowers

Karen Ashton
THE ESSENTIAL OILS GUIDE

Note

Top

Objective

Balancing

Associated Planet

Mercury

Extraction Method

Distillation

Main chemical constituents

Alcohols, Ester, Ketones, Sesquiterpene, Terpene

Aroma

Like Lavender: Clear, sweet and penetrating

Properties

Antidepressant, Analgesic, Cicatrisant, Expectorant, Nervine, Vulnerary

Karen Ashton
THE ESSENTIAL OILS GUIDE

Contra-Indications / Precautions

- Best avoided during first trimester of pregnancy
- Low blood pressure, may feel drowsy
- Not suitable for sedative actions (less relaxing than lavender)

Benefits Body Systems

Muscular system – aches & pains, stiffness
Respiratory system – Coughs, colds, flu, lung tonic, phlegm, sinus tonic
Skeletal system - rheumatism, stiff joints
The skin – dermatitis, scabies, wounds

Other healing properties

Rheumatism

Psychological / Emotional benefits

Refreshing, Tired mind

Karen Ashton
THE ESSENTIAL OILS GUIDE

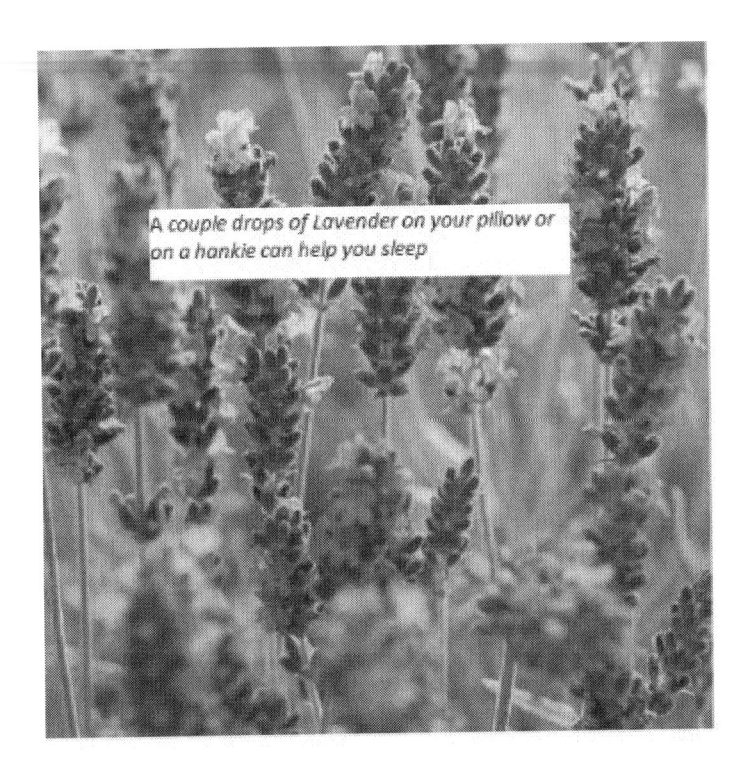

A couple drops of Lavender on your pillow or on a hankie can help you sleep

Karen Ashton
THE ESSENTIAL OILS GUIDE

Essential Oil Name

Lavender

Image

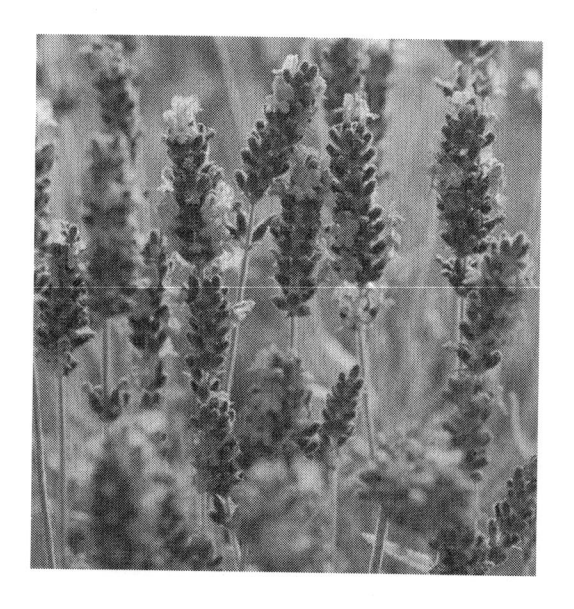

Botanical Name

Lavandula angustifolia

Plant

Flower

Karen Ashton
THE ESSENTIAL OILS GUIDE

Plant Family

Lamiaceae (Labiatae)

Category

Flower

Note

Middle

Objective

Relaxation, Stress relief

Associated Planet

Mercury

Extraction Method

Steam distillation

Main chemical constituents

Alcohols, Aldehydes, Esters, Ketones, Monoterpenes, Oxides, Sesquiterpenes

Karen Ashton
THE ESSENTIAL OILS GUIDE

Aroma

Floral & Light with a slight woody undertone

Properties

Analgesic, Anticonvulsive, Antidepressant, Antiphlogistic, Antirheumatic, Antiseptic, Antispasmodic, Antiviral, Bactericide, Carminative, Cholagogue, Cicatrisant, Cordial, Cytophalactic, Decongestant, Deodorant, Detoxicant, Diuretic, Emmenagogue, Fungicide, Hypotensive, Nervine, Restorative, Sedative, Splenetic, Sudorific, Vulnerary

Contra-Indications / Precautions

- May not be suitable for low blood pressure due to its drowsiness
- Best avoided in early months of pregnancy

Benefits Body Systems

Circulatory system – heart tonic, high blood pressure, hypertension, palpitations, poor circulation, varicose veins, white blood cells (helps to increase the production)
Digestive system – bile production, colic, flatulence, gall bladder stimulant, gastric secretion, nausea, sickness (travel), tonic to the liver, vomiting
Muscular system – aches, pains, spasms, sprains, strains

Karen Ashton
THE ESSENTIAL OILS GUIDE

Nervous system – epilepsy, headaches, migraine, nerve tonic, sciatica
Reproductive system – candida, dysmenorrhoea, labour pains & may help to speed up deliver, leucorrhoea, menstrual problems, periods (irregular, painful), PMS
Respiratory system – asthma, bronchitis, catarrh, colds, coughs, hay fever, laryngitis, throat (infections, sore), respiratory tract infections
Skeletal system – arthritis, rheumatism
The skin – abscesses, acne, alopecia, athlete's foot, bites, boils, bruises, burns, cell renewal, combination skin, dandruff, deodorant, diseases & disorders (Skin), eczema, fungal growth, hair tonic, hives, infections, infestations, itching, perspiration (induces), psoriasis, rejuvenating (skin), scarring, sebum balancing, spots, stretch marks, sunburn, warts, wounds
Urinary system – cystitis

Other healing properties

Can destroy micro-organisms, deodorant, headache, immune system stimulant, Inflammation, insect repellent, jet lag, rheumatism, tonic, toxins

Psychological / Emotional benefits

Anxiety, depression, emotions (tonic), frustration, hysteria, impatience, insomnia, nervous tension, panic, restlessness, shock, (helps to clear the) spleen (the seat of anger), stress, tantrum

Karen Ashton
THE ESSENTIAL OILS GUIDE

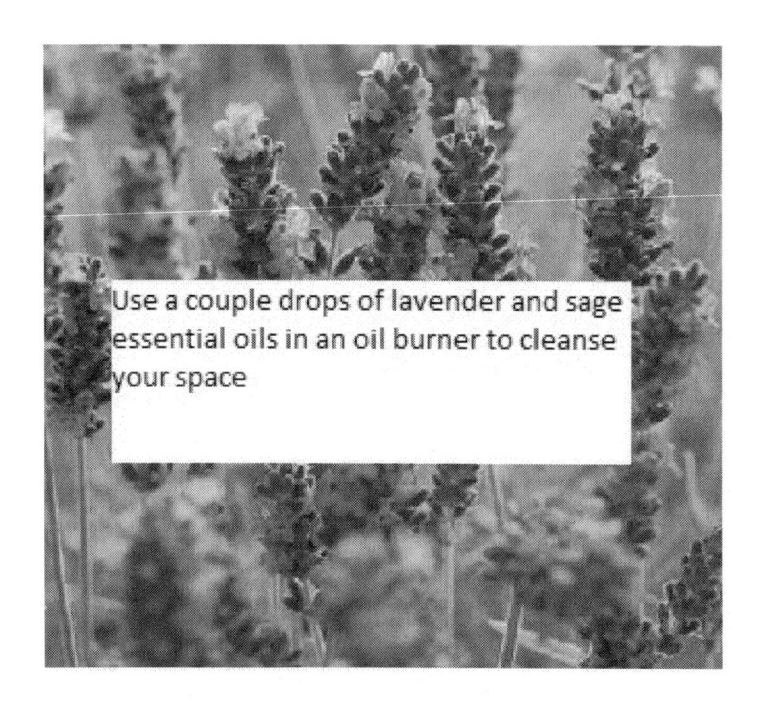

Use a couple drops of lavender and sage essential oils in an oil burner to cleanse your space

Karen Ashton
THE ESSENTIAL OILS GUIDE

Essential Oil Name

Lavender Spike

Image

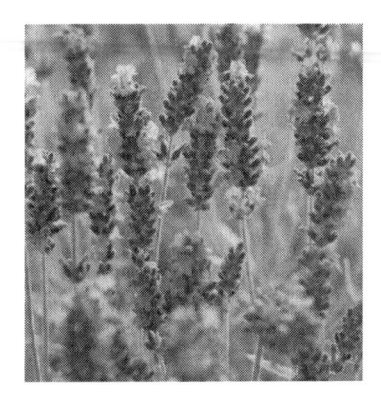

Botanical Name

Lavandula latifolia Medik

Plant

Flower

Plant Family

Lamiaceae (Labiatae)

Category

Flower

Karen Ashton
THE ESSENTIAL OILS GUIDE

Note

Top

Objective

Relaxation

Associated Planet

Mercury

Extraction Method

Steam distillation

Main chemical constituents

Alcohol, Ketones, Terpene

Aroma

Like Lavender but has a fresher, clearer aroma

Properties

Analgesic, Antidepressant, Antiseptic, Antiviral, Decongestant, Insecticide

Karen Ashton
THE ESSENTIAL OILS GUIDE

Contra-Indications / Precautions

- May be over-active to the central nervous system and cause palpitations if used in large amounts
- Best avoided in pregnancy

Benefits Body Systems

Muscular system – Pain
Nervous system – Headaches, relaxant
Respiratory system – Breathing (eases), Bronchitis, Catarrh, Laryngitis, Virus
Skeletal system – Rheumatism
The skin – Stings

Other healing properties

Balancing, Insect bites

Psychological / Emotional benefits

Alertness, Bereavement, Calming, Clears the mind, Hysteria, Irritability, Panic, Regret, Restlessness, Tranquiliser

Karen Ashton
THE ESSENTIAL OILS GUIDE

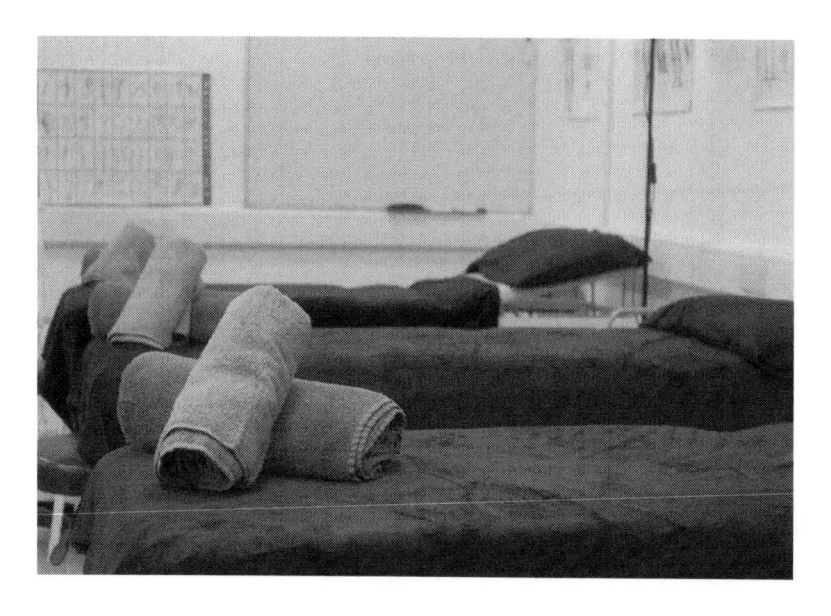

Training room @ www.holistictherapiestraining.co.uk

*"Wellness is the integration of the mind, body & soul.
It is the realisation that everything we do, think, feel &
believe, has an effect on our well-being!"*

Karen Ashton
THE ESSENTIAL OILS GUIDE

Essential Oil Name

Lemon

Image

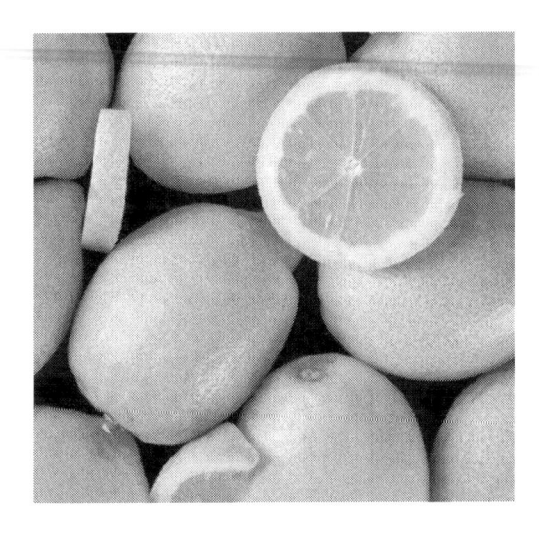

Botanical Name

Citrus limon

Plant

Fruit

Plant Family

Rutaceae

Karen Ashton
THE ESSENTIAL OILS GUIDE

Category

Citrus

Note

Top

Objective

Balancing

Associated Planet

Sun

Extraction Method

Expression / Steam distillation

Main chemical constituents

Alcohol, Aldehyde, Sesquiterpene, Terpene

Aroma

Fresh and sharp

Karen Ashton
THE ESSENTIAL OILS GUIDE

Properties

Antacid, Antisclerotic, Antiscorbutic, Antineuralgic, Antirheumatic, Antipruritic, Antiseptic, Astringent, Bactericide, Carminative, Cicatrisant, Depurative, Diuretic, Emollient, Escharotic, Febrifuge, Haemostatic, Hepatic, Hypoglycaemic, Hypotensive, Insecticide, Laxative, Stomachic, Tonic, Vermifuge

Contra-Indications / Precautions

- Hypersensitive skin

Benefits Body Systems

Circulatory system – anaemia, blood flow, high blood pressure, nose bleeds, tonic, varicose veins
Digestive system – acidity, constipation, decongestant to liver, pancreatic conditions, tonic
Endocrine system – diabetes
Nervous system – headaches, migraine, neuralgia
Respiratory system – Asthma, colds, coughs, fever, flu, hay fever, sore throat, temperature
Skeletal system – arthritis, rheumatism
The skin – brittle nails, capillaries (broken), cold sore, corns, dead skin cell removal, dull complexion, greasy hair, greasy skin, herpes, scar tissue, spots, stings, verruca's, warts, wounds
Urinary system – decongestant to kidneys

Other healing properties

Cellulite, cleansing action to the body, guilt, headache, helps the body to fight infectious diseases, insect bites, invigorates the immune system, rheumatism

Psychological / Emotional benefits

Clarity, cooling, jealousy, refreshing, regret

> **TIP:**
> If you are an Aromatherapist, do you pick oils for you or your client?

Karen Ashton
THE ESSENTIAL OILS GUIDE

Essential Oil Name

Lemongrass

Image

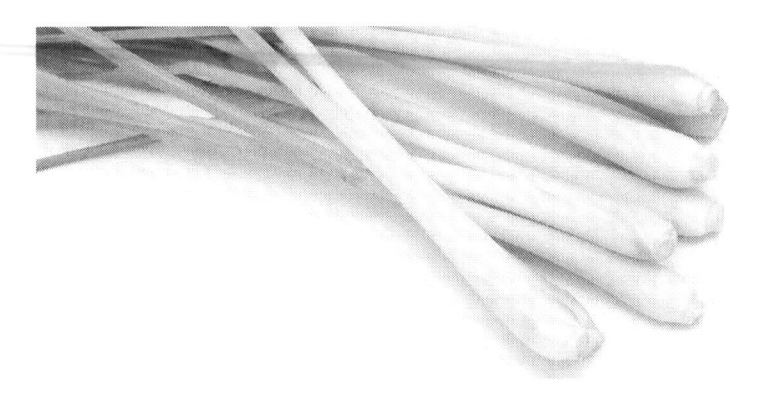

Botanical Name

Cymbopogon citratus

Plant

Grass

Plant Family

Poaceae (graminae)

Category

Citrus

Karen Ashton
THE ESSENTIAL OILS GUIDE

Note

Top

Objective

Balancing, Stress relief

Associated Planet

No associated planets

Extraction Method

Steam distillation

Main chemical constituents

Aldehydes, Ketones, Monoterpenes, Sesquiterpenes

Aroma

Sweet & Lemony, earthy, strong

Properties

Antidepressant, Antiseptic, Bactericide, Carminative, Deodorant, Digestive, Diuretic, Fungicide, Galactagogue, Insecticide, Prophylactic, Stimulant, Tonic

Karen Ashton
THE ESSENTIAL OILS GUIDE

Contra-Indications / Precautions

- Hypersensitive skin

Benefits Body Systems

Circulatory system – stimulates circulation
Digestive system – appetite (boosts), colitis, digestive muscles, flatulence, gastro-enteritis, indigestion, liver tonic, stimulant, tonic
Endocrine system – glandular secretions
Lymphatic system – cellulite, fluid retention
Muscular system – aches, lactic acid (helps to eliminate), pains, suppleness, tired legs, toning
Nervous system – headaches, parasympathetic nerve boost
Respiratory system – fevers, laryngitis, sore throats, upper respiratory tract infections
The skin – acne, athlete's foot, cellulite, fungal infections, open pores, oily skin, loose skin tone

Other healing properties

A good all-round tonic for the body, a boost to the immune system, aids healing, headache, jet lag, fatigue, insect repellent, resists / destroys micro-organisms & bacteria

Psychological / Emotional benefits

Clears the head, depression, energising, exhaustion, movement (helps to get things moving), nervous tension, reviving, spirit lifting, stimulating, stress, uplifting

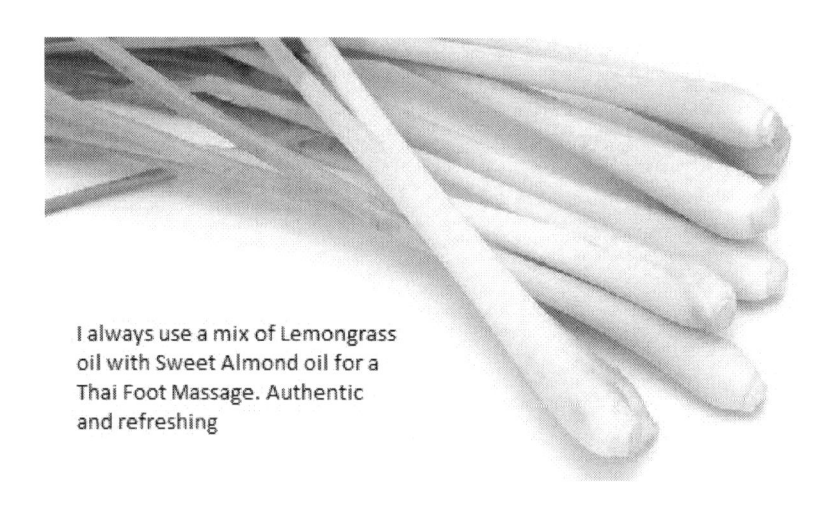

I always use a mix of Lemongrass oil with Sweet Almond oil for a Thai Foot Massage. Authentic and refreshing

Essential Oil Name

Mandarin

Image

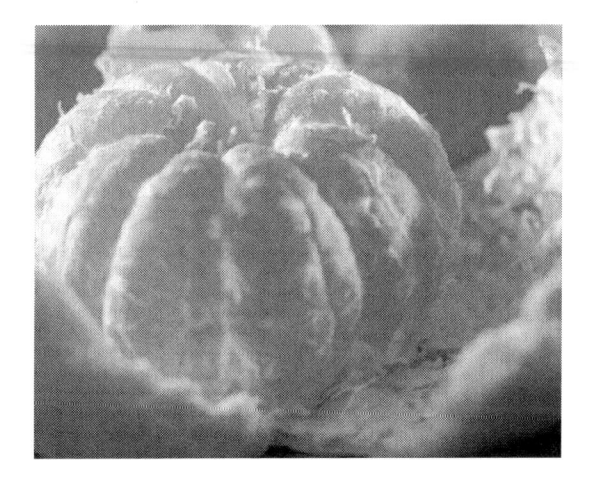

Botanical Name

Citrus nobilis Lour

Plant

Fruit

Plant Family

Rutaceae

Karen Ashton
THE ESSENTIAL OILS GUIDE

Category

Citrus

Note

Top / Middle

Objective

Uplift/Stimulation

Associated Planet

Sun

Extraction Method

Expression

Main chemical constituents

Alcohol, Aldehyde, Ester, Terpene

Aroma

Sweet & tangy, with slight floral undertone

Karen Ashton
THE ESSENTIAL OILS GUIDE

Properties

Antispasmodic, Cholagogue, Cytophalactic, Digestive, Emollient, Sedative, Tonic

Contra-Indications / Precautions

- Could be phototoxic, avoid if going in direct sunlight

Benefits Body Systems

Digestive system – Appetite stimulant, Bile secretion, Calming, Fat breakdown, Gas expulsion, Liver stimulant, Metabolic processes, Morning sickness, Tonic
Reproductive system – PMT
The skin – Scarring, Stretch marks

Other healing properties

Fragile, suitable for children and pregnancy in milder doses

Psychological / Emotional benefits

Anxiety, Depression, Revitalising, Strengthening, Tantrums, Uplifting

Karen Ashton
THE ESSENTIAL OILS GUIDE

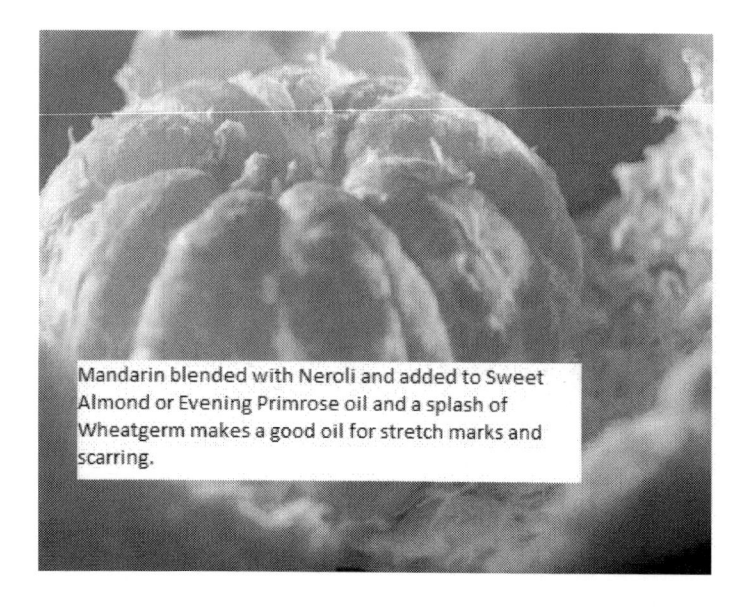

Mandarin blended with Neroli and added to Sweet Almond or Evening Primrose oil and a splash of Wheatgerm makes a good oil for stretch marks and scarring.

Karen Ashton
THE ESSENTIAL OILS GUIDE

Essential Oil Name

Marjoram

Image

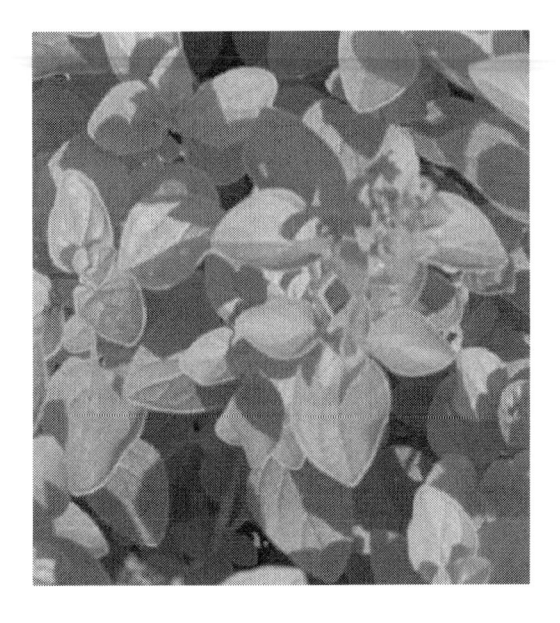

Botanical Name

Origanum majorana

Plant

Herb

Plant Family

Lamiaceae (Labiatae)

Category

Herb

Note

Middle

Objective

Relaxation, Stress relief

Associated Planet

Mercury

Extraction Method

Steam distillation

Main chemical constituents

Alcohols, Aldehydes, Esters, Monoterpenes, Phenols, Sesquiterpenes

Karen Ashton
THE ESSENTIAL OILS GUIDE

Aroma

Warm & slightly spicy, woody

Properties

Analgesic, Anaphrodisiac, Antiseptic, Antispasmodic, Carminative, Cephalic, Cordial, Digestive, Emmenagogue, Expectorant, Hypotensive, Laxative, Nervine, Restorative, Sedative, Tonic, Vulnerary

Contra-Indications / Precautions

- Can cause drowsiness if overused
- Pregnancy

Benefits Body Systems

Circulatory system – arteries, blood flow, blood vessels (relaxes), capillaries, chilblains, circulation, heart tonic, high blood pressure, low body temperature
Digestive system – colic, constipation, diarrhoea, flatulence, indigestion, sickness, soothing, stimulant, stomach cramps, toxin clearing
Muscular system – cramp, muscle aches, pains & strains, warming
Nervous system – epilepsy, headaches, migraines, neuralgia, sensation (could quell), tonic, vertigo

Reproductive system – amenorrhoea, dysmenorrhoea, leucorrhoea, menstrual cycle regulation, PMT, period pain, sexual desire (could quell)
Respiratory system – asthma, bronchitis, chest infections, colds, congestion, cough (tickly), flu, sinusitis, viruses
Skeletal system – arthritis, joint stiffness & cold, rheumatic aches & pains, sprains, swollen joints
The skin – bruises, wounds

Other healing properties

Good health, after sport / exercise, headache, insomnia, rheumatism

Psychological / Emotional benefits
Anxiety, bereavement, exhaustion, grief, guilt, hysteria, insomnia, jealousy, loneliness, restlessness, shock, stress, worry

> **TIP:**
> For Aromatherapists, remember to consider contra-indications that you have as well as your clients. i.e., if you are pregnant, you will not be able to use oils on clients that are unsuitable for pregnancy, as you will absorb the oils as well as your client!

Karen Ashton
THE ESSENTIAL OILS GUIDE

Essential Oil Name

Myrrh

Image

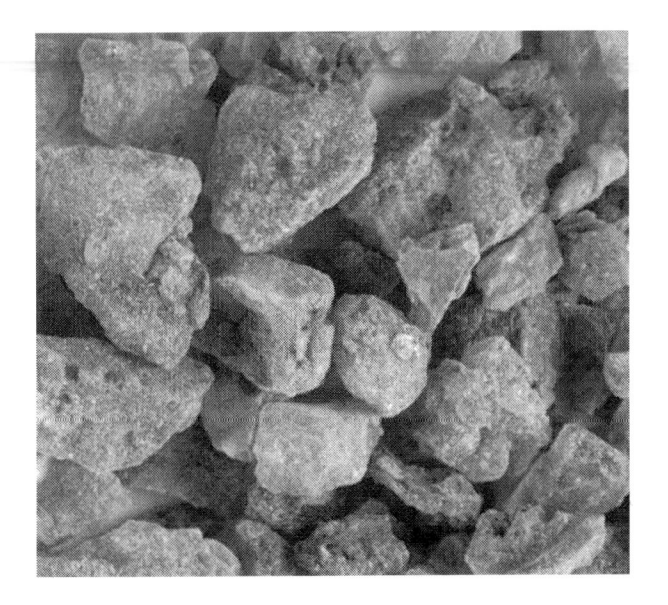

Botanical Name

Commiphora myrrha

Plant

Resin

Karen Ashton
THE ESSENTIAL OILS GUIDE

Plant Family

Burseraceae

Category

Resin

Note

Base

Objective

Balancing

Associated Planet

Sun

Extraction Method

Distillation

Main chemical constituents

Acid, Aldehyde, Phenol, Sesquiterpene, Terpene

Aroma

Smokey, Musty

Karen Ashton
THE ESSENTIAL OILS GUIDE

Properties

Antiseptic, Antimicrobial, Antiphlogistic, Astringent, Balsamic, Deodorant, Carminative, Disinfectant, Diuretic, Emmenagogue, Expectorant, Fungicide, Stimulant, Stomachic, Sudorific, Tonic, Uterine, Vulnerary

Contra-Indications / Precautions

- Avoid during pregnancy

Benefits Body Systems

Circulatory system – pulmonary complaints, stimulates white blood corpuscles
Digestive system – acidity, appetite stimulant, bad breath, diarrhoea, flatulence, gastric fermentation, gum disorder, mouth disorders, mucus, piles, tonic
Reproductive system – irregular periods, leucorrhoea, thrush, cleansing to the womb
Respiration system – bronchitis, catarrh, colds, coughs, glandular fever, pharyngitis, sore throats, virus
The skin – athletes' foot, boils, chapped skin, eczema weeping, hives, inflammation, moist skin conditions, sores, tissue degeneration, ulcers, weeping wounds

Other healing properties

Boosts the immune system, cleansing, helps the body to recover from disease, inflammation

Psychological / Emotional benefits

Apathy, bereavement, cooling on the emotions, incentive, weakness

> I'm old school when it comes to the ingestion of essential oils. My training and research confirmed you are not allowed to consult clients to ingest oils unless you have received the relevant training.

Karen Ashton
THE ESSENTIAL OILS GUIDE

Essential Oil Name

Neroli

Image

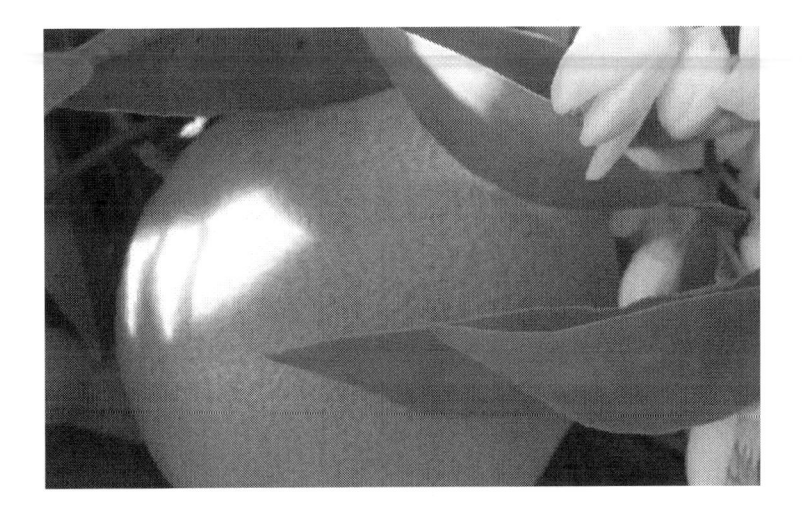

Botanical Name

Citrus aurantium

Plant

Flowers

Plant Family

Ruttaceae

Karen Ashton
THE ESSENTIAL OILS GUIDE

Category

Flower

Note

Base

Objective

Relaxation, Stress relief

Associated Planet

Sun

Extraction Method

Steam distillation

Main chemical constituents

Acids, Alcohols, Esters, Indole, Ketones, Monoterpenes

Aroma

Floral

Karen Ashton
THE ESSENTIAL OILS GUIDE

Properties

Antidepressant, Antiseptic, Antispasmodic, Aphrodisiac, Bactericide, Carminative, Cordial, Cytophalactic, Deodorant, Digestive, Emollient, Sedative, Tonic

Contra-Indications / Precautions

- May affect concentration as deeply relaxing
- Phototoxic - can cause skin sensitivity

Benefits Body Systems

Circulatory system – blood cleansing, cell regenerator, circulation, palpitations, thread veins, tonic to the heart
Digestive system – calming on the intestines, colitis, diarrhoea, flatulence, indigestion
Nervous system – headache, neuralgia, sympathetic nervous system relaxant, tonic, vertigo
Reproductive system – aphrodisiac, menopausal problems, PMT, sexual problems, tonic to the uterus
The skin – cell regeneration, combination skin, dermatitis, dry skin, eczema, elasticity, mature, psoriasis, scarring, sensitive skin, stretch marks, X-rays (can help protect skin during), wrinkles

Other healing properties

Can destroy / inhibit growth of micro-organisms, headache, helps to regenerate cells

Karen Ashton
THE ESSENTIAL OILS GUIDE

Psychological / Emotional benefits

Anger, anxiety, bereavement, claustrophobia, depression, euphoric, hypnotic, hysteria, insomnia, irritability, negativity, (helps to instil a feeling of) peace, restlessness, shock, stress, tearfulness

> **TIP:**
> For Pregnancy, citrus oils are relatively safe oils to use

Karen Ashton
THE ESSENTIAL OILS GUIDE

Essential Oil Name

Orange (Sweet)

Image

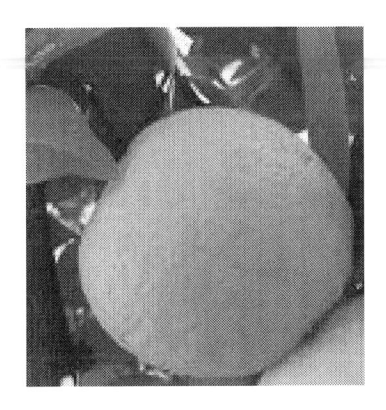

Botanical Name

Citrus sinensis

Plant

Fruit

Plant Family

Rutaceae

Category

Citrus

Karen Ashton
THE ESSENTIAL OILS GUIDE

Note

Top

Objective

Relaxation

Associated Planet

Sun

Extraction Method

Expression

Main chemical constituents

Alcohol, Aldehyde, Ester, Terpene

Aroma

Refreshing and zesty

Properties

Antidepressant, Antiseptic, Antispasmodic, Carminative, Digestive, Febrifuge, Sedative, Stomachic, Tonic

Karen Ashton
THE ESSENTIAL OILS GUIDE

Contra-Indications / Precautions

- May irritate sensitive skin if used in excess
- Phototoxic

Benefits Body Systems

Circulatory system – Cholesterol levels
Digestive system – Appetite stimulant, Bile stimulant, Calming, Constipation, Diarrhoea, Digestion of fats, Gastric complaints, Vitamin C absorption
Muscular system – Painful & sore muscles
Respiration system – Bronchitis, Colds, Fever
Skeletal system – Rickety bones
The skin – Collagen formation, Congestion, Dermatitis, Dry Skin, Growth & repair of tissue, Sweating, Tonic, Toxins, Wrinkles

Other healing properties

Viral

Psychological / Emotional benefits

Anger, Anxiety, Butterflies in stomach, Depression, Frustration, Grief, Insomnia, irritability, Negativity, Nervous states, Sadness

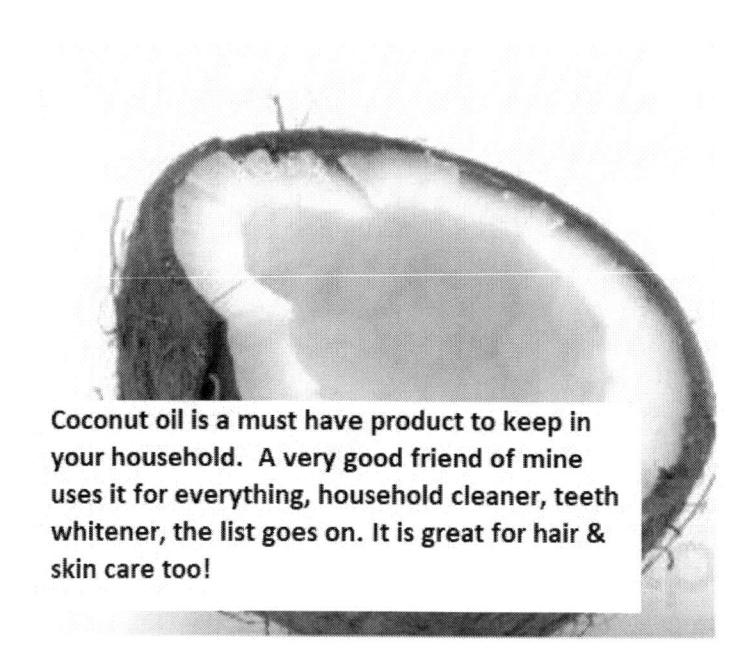

Coconut oil is a must have product to keep in your household. A very good friend of mine uses it for everything, household cleaner, teeth whitener, the list goes on. It is great for hair & skin care too!

Karen Ashton
THE ESSENTIAL OILS GUIDE

Essential Oil Name

Patchouli

Image

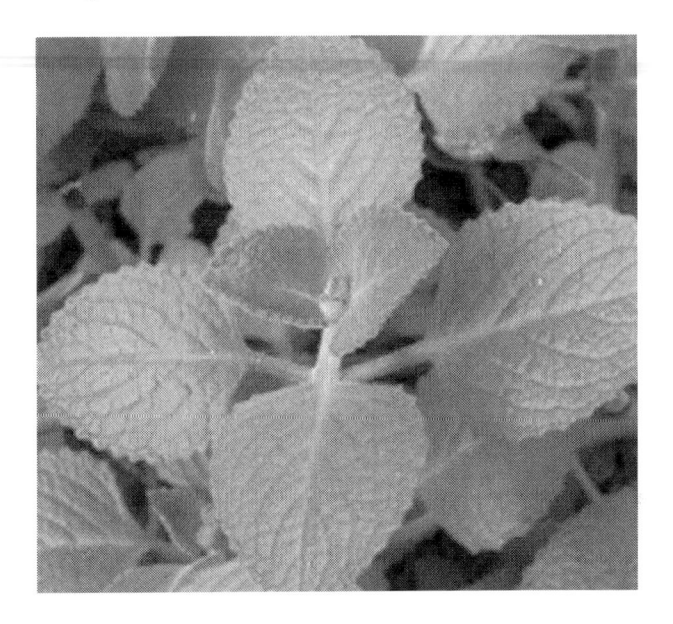

Botanical Name

Pogostemon cablin Benth

Plant

Leaves

Plant Family

Lamiaceae (Labiatae)

Category

Exotic

Note

Base

Objective

Balancing, Stress relief

Associated Planet

Sun

Extraction Method

Steam distillation

Main chemical constituents

Alcohols, Ketones, Oxides, Monoterpenes, Sesquiterpenes

Karen Ashton
THE ESSENTIAL OILS GUIDE

Aroma

Sweet, earthy, exotic, musky

Properties

Antidepressant, Antimicrobial, Antiphlogistic, Antiseptic, Aphrodisiac, Astringent, Cicatrisant, Cytophalactic, Deodorant, Diuretic, Febrifuge, Fungicide, Insecticide, Sedative, Tonic

Contra-Indications / Precautions

- Can be sedative as well as stimulating so care taken on dosages
- Can cause loss of appetite
- Aroma can be overpowering for some people

Benefits Body Systems

Circulatory system – fever, varicose veins
Digestive system – appetite (curbs), constipation, diarrhoea, diuretic
Lymphatic system – fluid retention
Nervous system – balancing on the central nervous system
Reproductive system – Aphrodisiac, tonic to the uterus
Respiratory system – viruses
The skin – acne, athlete's foot, cells, cellulite, combination skin, cracked skin, dandruff, deodorising,

dry skin, eczema, fungal, inflammation, rough/cracked skin, scalp disorders, scar tissue, sebum (helps to stimulate the production, sores, sweating, tissue regeneration, wounds (incl., weeping)
Urinary system – cystitis

Other healing properties

Could help with weight reduction as it curbs appetite and helps to tone loose skin from dieting, Immune system tonic, Insect / Snake bites

Psychological / Emotional benefits

Anxiety, balancing, clarification, debility, depression, nervous exhaustion, grounding, indecision, insecurity, lethargy, libido, mood swings, objective, stress, (helps to sharpen the) wits

Karen Ashton
THE ESSENTIAL OILS GUIDE

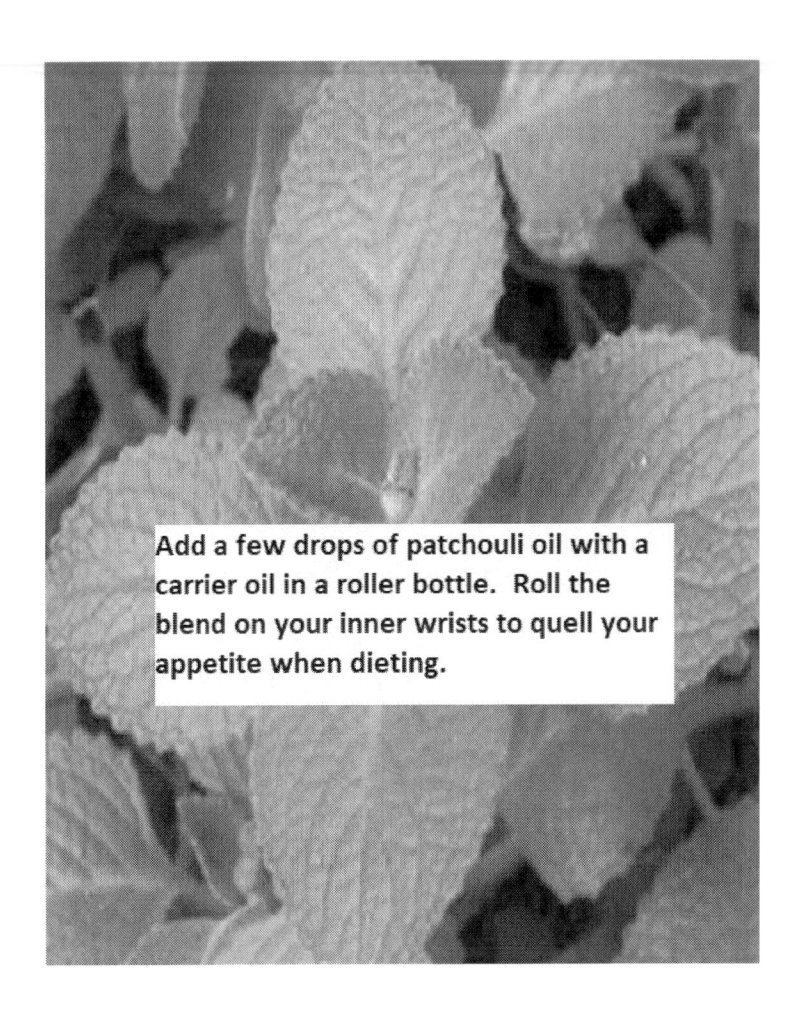

Add a few drops of patchouli oil with a carrier oil in a roller bottle. Roll the blend on your inner wrists to quell your appetite when dieting.

Karen Ashton
THE ESSENTIAL OILS GUIDE

Essential Oil Name

Peppermint

Image

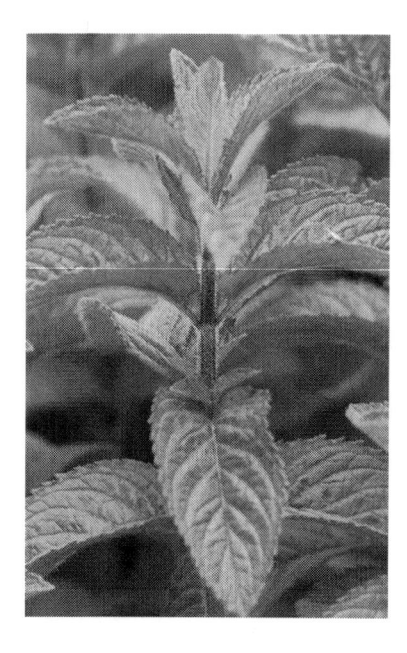

Botanical Name

Mentha x piperita

Plant

Herb

Karen Ashton
THE ESSENTIAL OILS GUIDE

Plant Family

Lamiaceae (Labiatae)

Category

Herb

Note

Top

Objective

Balancing

Associated Planet

Venus

Extraction Method

Distillation

Main chemical constituents

Alcohol, Ester, Ketone, Phenol, Terpene

Aroma

Sharp, menthol and strong

Karen Ashton
THE ESSENTIAL OILS GUIDE

Properties

Anaesthetic, Analgesic, Antidontalgic, Antigalactagogue, Antiphlogistic, Antiseptic, Antispasmodic, Astringent, Carminative, Cephalic, Cholagogue, Cordial, Decongestant, Emmenagogue, Expectorant, Febrifuge, Hepatic, Nervine, Stimulant, Stomachic, Sudorific, Vasoconstrictor, Vermifuge

Contra-Indications / Precautions

- Excessive use can be too overwhelming
- Could cause skin irritation
- Could irritate mucous membranes
- Avoid if pregnant
- Avoid if nursing as could discourage milk production
- May antidote homeopathic remedies

Benefits Body Systems

Circulatory system – Anaemia, Tonic
Digestive system – Acute digestive conditions, Colic, Constipation, Diarrhoea, Flatulence, Food poisoning, Gall stones, Halitosis, Indigestion, Liver disorder, Nausea, Travel sickness, Vomiting
Muscular system – Aches, Relaxing on stomach muscles
Nervous system – Headaches, Migraines, Neuralgia, Toothache

Karen Ashton
THE ESSENTIAL OILS GUIDE

Reproductive system – Irregular periods, Mastitis, Painful periods
Respiratory system – Asthma, Bronchitis, Cholera, Colds, Dry coughs, Fevers, Mucous, Pneumonia, Sinus congestion, Sinusitis, Tuberculosis
Skeletal system – Rheumatism
The skin – Blackheads, Capillary constriction, Congestion of toxins, Dermatitis, Greasy hair, Greasy skin, Inflammation, Itching, Perspiration stimulant, Pruritis, Ringworm, Scabies, Sunburn
Urinary system – Kidney disorders

Other healing properties

Aching feet, Balancing heat, Dizziness, Fainting, Fatigue, Headache, Insect bites, Jet lag, numbness in limbs, Pain relief, Rheumatism

Psychological / Emotional benefits

Exhaustion, Impatience, Indecision, Irritability, Shock, Tonic to the mind, Vertigo

Karen Ashton
THE ESSENTIAL OILS GUIDE

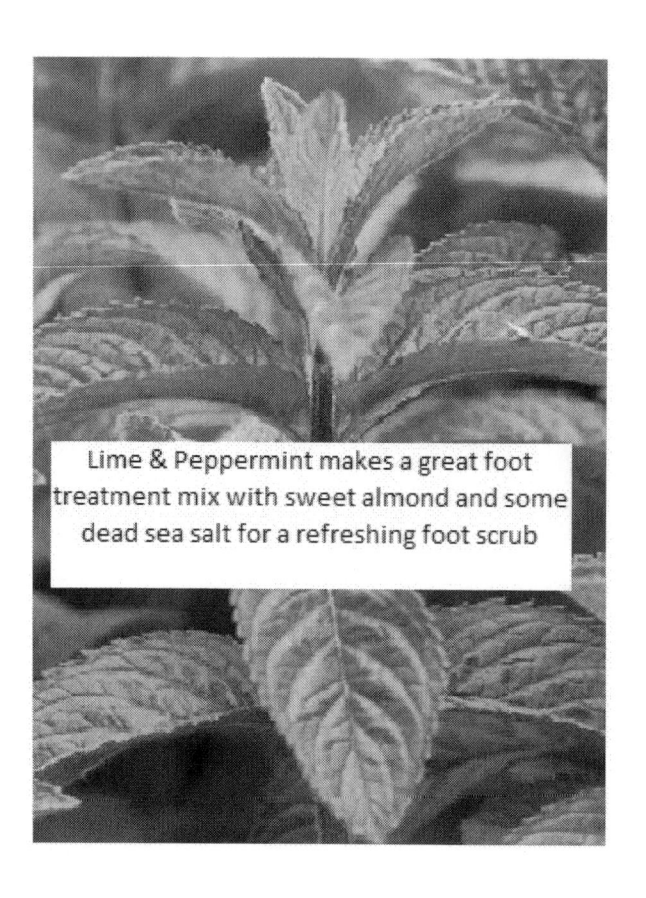

Lime & Peppermint makes a great foot treatment mix with sweet almond and some dead sea salt for a refreshing foot scrub

Karen Ashton
THE ESSENTIAL OILS GUIDE

Essential Oil Name

Petitgrain

Image

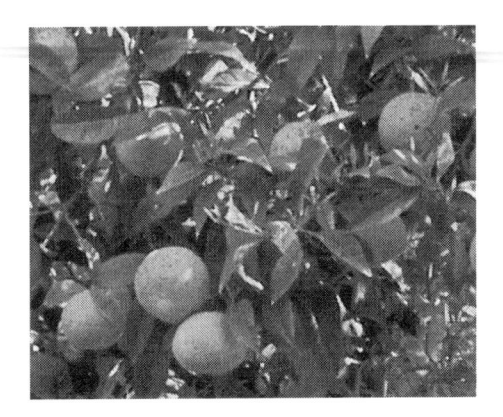

Botanical Name

Citrus aurantium

Plant

Leaves

Plant Family

Ruttaceae

Karen Ashton
THE ESSENTIAL OILS GUIDE

Category

Tree

Note

Top

Objective

Relaxation, Stress relief

Associated Planet

Sun

Extraction Method

Steam distillation

Main chemical constituents

Alcohols, Esters, Monoterpenes

Aroma

Floral, woody, sweet & fresh

Karen Ashton
THE ESSENTIAL OILS GUIDE

Properties

Antidepressant, Antiseptic, Antispasmodic, Deodorant, Sedative

Contra-Indications / Precautions

No known precautions

Benefits Body Systems

Circulatory system – rapid heartbeat
Digestive system – flatulence, Indigestion
Muscular system – muscle spasms
Nervous system – sedative to the nervous system
Reproductive system – PMS
Respiratory system – breathlessness
The skin – acne, congested skin, dry skin, oily skin, perspiration (excessive)

Other healing properties

Helps to slow the body down

Psychological / Emotional benefits

Anger, anxiety, depression, insomnia, irritability, nervous exhaustion, panic, reassurance when feeling down, refreshing to the mind, relaxing, soothing, stress

Karen Ashton
THE ESSENTIAL OILS GUIDE

Essential Oil Name

Rose

Image

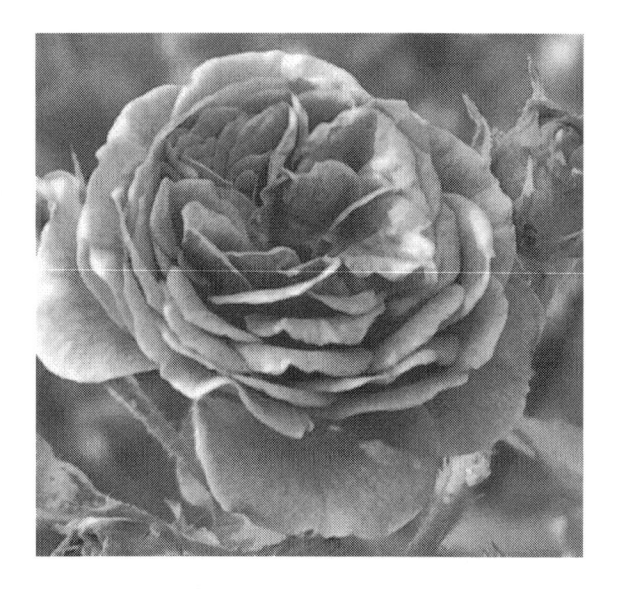

Botanical Name

Rose Damask - Rosa damascene

Rose Cabbage - Rosa centifolia

Plant

flowers

Karen Ashton
THE ESSENTIAL OILS GUIDE

Plant Family

Rosaceae

Category

Flower

Note

Base

Objective

Balancing, Stress relief

Associated Planet

Venus

Extraction Method

Steam distillation

Main chemical constituents

Alcohols, Esters, Oxides, Monoterpenes

Aroma

Deep, Floral, Sweet & rich

Karen Ashton
THE ESSENTIAL OILS GUIDE

Properties

Antidepressant, Antiphlogistic, Antiseptic, Antispasmodic, Aphrodisiac, Bactericide, Cholagogue, Depurative, Diuretic, Emmenagogue, Haemostatic, Hepatic, Laxative, Sedative, Splenetic, Stomachic, Tonic

Contra-Indications / Precautions

- Pregnancy
- Highly concentrated so use sparingly

Benefits Body Systems

Circulatory system – 'slows' bleeding, circulation, palpitations, thread veins, tonic to the circulatory
Digestive system – appetite regulator, balance and strengthen the stomach, bile production, constipation, gall bladder & liver congestion, nausea, tonic, vomiting
Endocrine system – Helps to release the happy hormone 'dopamine'
Muscular system - aches
Nervous system – headaches
Reproductive system – aphrodisiac, frigidity, impotence, leucorrhoea, menopause, menstrual cycle, PMT, reproductive problems, secretions (male & female), sexual problems, tonic to the womb
Respiratory system – coughs, hay fever, sore throat
The skin – ageing skin, all skin types, allergies, combination skin, dermatitis, dry skin, eczema, healing,

hives, inflammation, mature skin, rosacea, scar tissue, sensitive skin, shingles, tonic, soothing

Other healing properties

Hangovers, headache, helps to remove toxins

Psychological / Emotional benefits

Anxiety, depression, fear, grief, guilt, insomnia, jealousy, panic, (female) positivity oil, regret, resentment, soothing, stress, tantrum, 'nervous' tension, uplifting, upsets emotional

> **TIP**
> Castor Oil is said to help with hair growth. We tried it on my son when he had a rather short hair cut in his teenage years and wasn't happy with it. I've also known people to put it on their eyebrows to help with growing them back to reshape and on eyelashes (carefully!) to help their eyelashes to grow longer.

Karen Ashton
THE ESSENTIAL OILS GUIDE

Essential Oil Name

Rosemary

Image

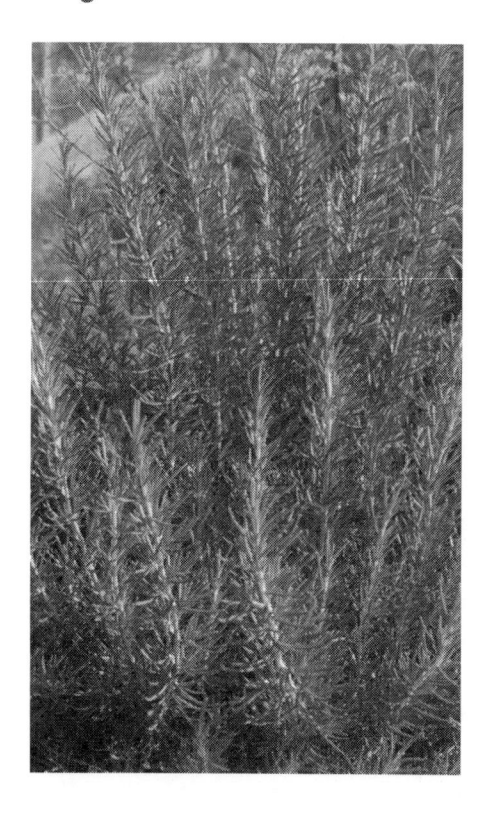

Botanical Name

Rosmarinus officinalis

Karen Ashton
THE ESSENTIAL OILS GUIDE

Plant

Herb

Plant Family

Lamiaceae (Labiatae)

Category

Herb

Note

Middle

Objective

Balancing, Stress relief

Associated Planet

Sun

Extraction Method

Distillation

Karen Ashton
THE ESSENTIAL OILS GUIDE

Main chemical constituents

Alcohol, Aldehyde, Ester, Camphene, Camphor, Ketone, Sesquiterpene, Terpene,

Aroma

Strong, Herbal

Properties

Analgesic, Antidepressant, Antirheumatic, Antiseptic, Antispasmodic, Astringent, Carminative, Cephalic, Cholagogue, Cicatrisant, Cordial, Digestive, Diuretic, Emmenagogue, Hepatic, Hypertensive, Nervine, Resolvent, Stimulant, Stomachic, Sudorific, Tonic, Vulnerary

Contra-Indications / Precautions

- Epilepsy
- High blood pressure
- Pregnancy
- May antidote homeopathic remedies

Karen Ashton
THE ESSENTIAL OILS GUIDE

Benefits Body Systems

Circulatory system – anaemia, blood pressure low, circulation, tonic to the heart
Digestive system – catarrh, colitis, flatulence, gall stones, indigestion, liver decongestant, stomach pains
Lymphatic system – oedema, water retention
Muscular system – aches, sprains
Nervous system –energise the brain, headache, migraine, nerve stimulant, neuralgia, sciatica, vertigo
Reproductive system – candida, menstrual cramps, regulate periods
Respiratory system – asthma, bronchitis, colds, flu, tonic to the lungs
Skeletal system – arthritis, rheumatic pain
The skin – cellulite, congestion, dandruff, hair growth, lice, sagging skin, scalp disorders, swelling, toning, watery

Other healing properties

Fatigue, headache, pain relief, revives the senses, rheumatic pain

Psychological / Emotional benefits

Clears the head, depression, dullness, exhaustion, indecision, lethargy, loneliness, memory, mental strain, sadness, self-control, strengthening in times of weakness & exhaustion

Karen Ashton
THE ESSENTIAL OILS GUIDE

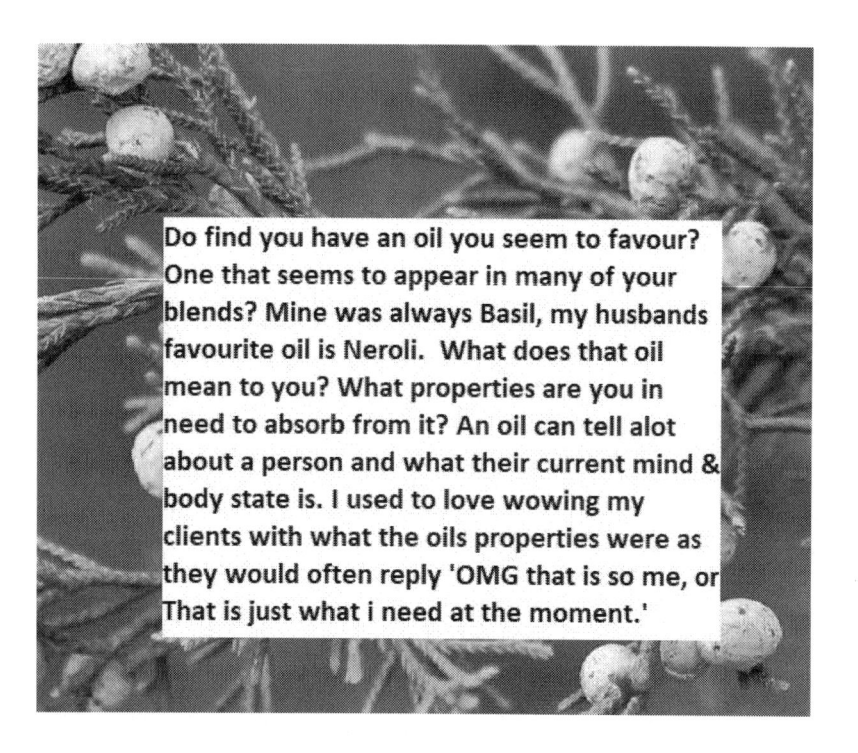

Do find you have an oil you seem to favour? One that seems to appear in many of your blends? Mine was always Basil, my husbands favourite oil is Neroli. What does that oil mean to you? What properties are you in need to absorb from it? An oil can tell alot about a person and what their current mind & body state is. I used to love wowing my clients with what the oils properties were as they would often reply 'OMG that is so me, or That is just what i need at the moment.'

Karen Ashton
THE ESSENTIAL OILS GUIDE

Essential Oil Name

Sandalwood

Image

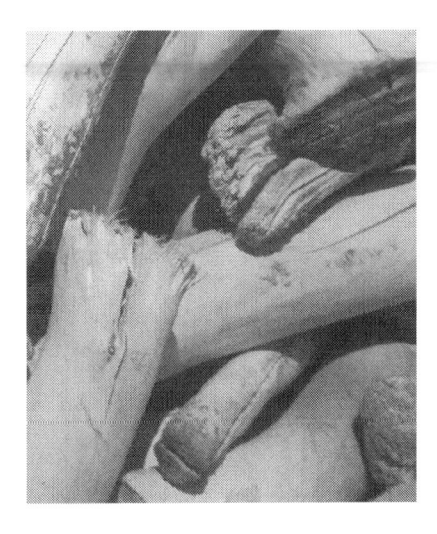

Botanical Name

Santalum album

Plant

Wood

Plant Family

Santalaceae

Karen Ashton
THE ESSENTIAL OILS GUIDE

Category

Exotic

Note

Base

Objective

Relaxation, Stress relief

Associated Planet

No known associated planet

Extraction Method

Distillation

Main chemical constituents

Alcohol, Aldehyde, Sesquiterpene

Aroma

Woody, Exotic, Subtle

Karen Ashton
THE ESSENTIAL OILS GUIDE

Properties

Antiphlogistic, Antiseptic, Antispasmodic, Aphrodisiac, Astringent, Bechic, Carminative, Diuretic, Emollient, Expectorant, Sedative, Tonic

Contra-Indications / Precautions

- It is best to avoid during depression in case of mood lowering
- Strong aphrodisiac

Benefits Body Systems

Circulatory system – heartburn
Digestive system – diarrhoea, nausea
Reproductive system – aphrodisiac, cleansing to the sexual organs, cystitis, frigidity, impotence, STD's
Respiratory system – bronchitis, catarrh, chest infections, coughs, lung infections, sore throats
The skin – acne, ageing skin, balancing, boils, dehydration, dry skin, eczema, inflammation, itching, mature skin, psoriasis, scalp tonic, softening, sunburn, wounds
Urinary system – cystitis, tonic to the kidneys

Other healing properties

Anti-inflammatory, boosts the immune system

Karen Ashton
THE ESSENTIAL OILS GUIDE

Psychological / Emotional benefits

Acceptance, anxiety, claustrophobia, cut ties with the past, impatience, insecurity, insomnia, jealousy, nervous tension, obsessional states, peace, regret, relaxing, sedative, stress, well-being, worry

> **TIP:**
> Try to vary the oils used for yourself or your clients as your body can become used to the oils so may not have as powerful an effect.

Karen Ashton
THE ESSENTIAL OILS GUIDE

Essential Oil Name

Tea Tree

Image

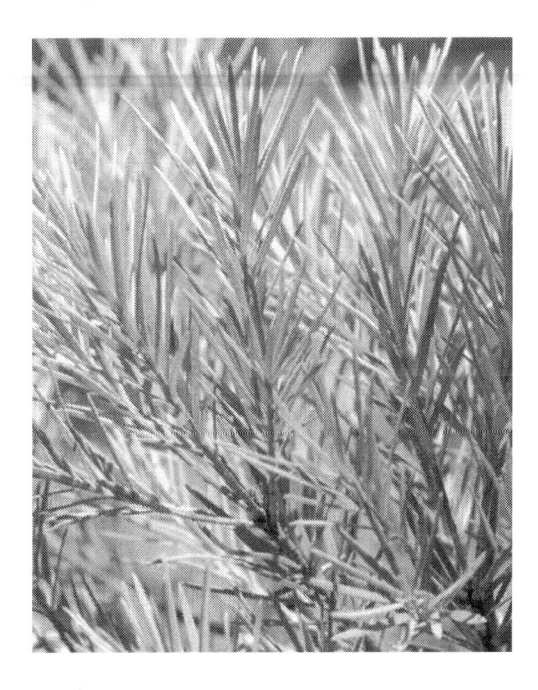

Botanical Name

Melaleuca alternifolia Cheel

Plant

Leaves

Karen Ashton
THE ESSENTIAL OILS GUIDE

Plant Family

Myrtaceae

Category

Tree

Note

Top

Objective

Uplift/Stimulation

Associated Planet

No known associated planets

Extraction Method

Distillation

Main chemical constituents

Alcohol, Cymene, Ketone, Pinene, Terpene

Aroma

Fresh, clean, strong

Karen Ashton
THE ESSENTIAL OILS GUIDE

Properties

Antibiotic, Antipruritic, Antiseptic, Antiviral, Bactericide, Balsamic, Cicatrisant, Cordial, Expectorant, Fungicide, Insecticide, Stimulant, Sudorific

Contra-Indications / Precautions

- Hypersensitive skin

Benefits Body Systems

Digestive system – inflammatory conditions
Lymphatic system –toxins
Muscular system - aches
Reproductive system – candida
Respiratory system – bronchitis, catarrh, colds, flu, sinusitis, sore throat
The skin – athlete's foot, blemishes, burns, chicken pox, cleansing, cold sores, congestion, dandruff, dry scalp, head lice, pruritis, pus, ringworm, scalp tonic, scarring, shingles, sores, spots, sunburn, verruca's, warts, wounds
Urinary system – cystitis, UTI

Other healing properties

Boost the immune system to fight off infections, can help to fortify the body in preparation for surgery, convalescence, insect bites

Psychological / Emotional benefits

Refreshing, revitalising, shock (incl., post-operative)

Karen Ashton
THE ESSENTIAL OILS GUIDE

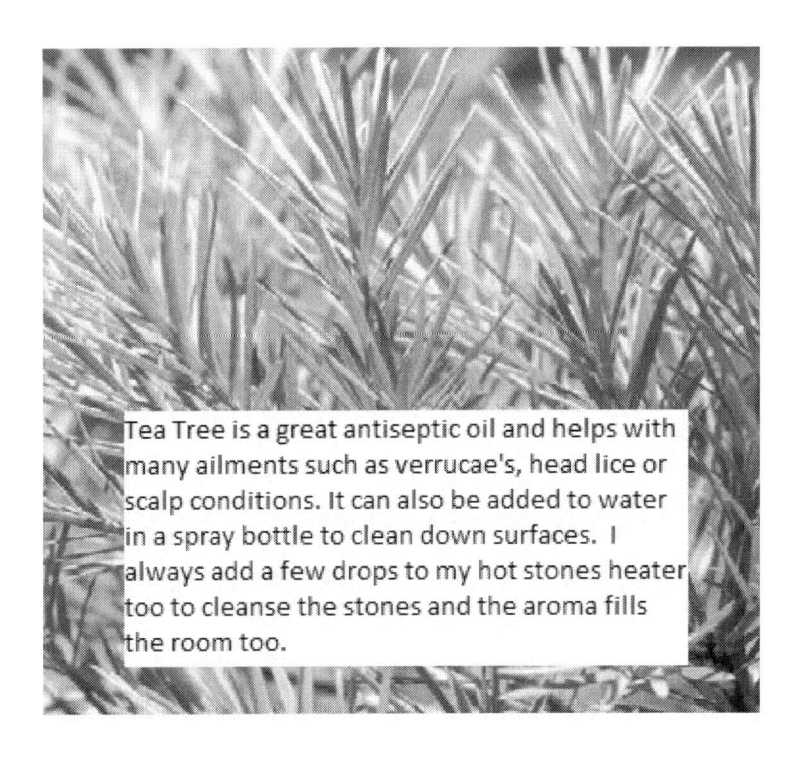

Tea Tree is a great antiseptic oil and helps with many ailments such as verrucae's, head lice or scalp conditions. It can also be added to water in a spray bottle to clean down surfaces. I always add a few drops to my hot stones heater too to cleanse the stones and the aroma fills the room too.

Essential Oil Name

Thyme

Image

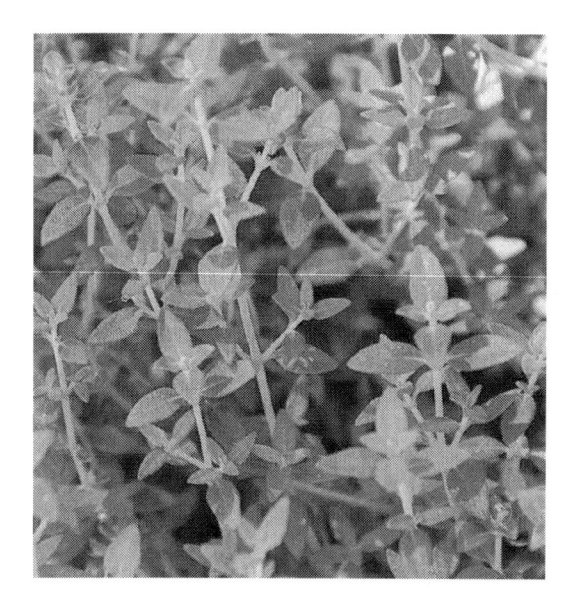

Botanical Name

Thymus vulgaris

Plant

Herb

Karen Ashton
THE ESSENTIAL OILS GUIDE

Plant Family

Lamiaceae (Labiatae)

Category

Herb

Note

Top / Middle

Objective

Uplift/Stimulation

Associated Planet

Venus

Extraction Method

Distillation

Main chemical constituents

Alcohol, Borneol, Carvacrol, Cymene, Phenol, Sesquiterpene, Terpene

Karen Ashton
THE ESSENTIAL OILS GUIDE

Aroma

Sweet, herbal

Properties

Antimicrobe, Antirheumatic, Antiseptic, Antispasmodic, Antiputrefactive, Antivenomous, Aperitif, Aphrodisiac, Bactericide, Bechic, Cardiac, Carminative, Cicatrisant, Diuretic, Emmenagogue, Expectorant, Hypertensive, Insecticide, Stimulant, Tonic, Vermifuge

Contra-Indications / Precautions

- Can be toxic in prolonged use
- Better for inhalation as opposed to bathing or massage use
- Can be an irritant to the skin
- High blood pressure
- Pregnancy

Benefits Body Systems

Circulatory system –circulation, low blood pressure, nose bleeds
Digestive system – dyspepsia, gastric complaints, stimulant to the digestive system, wind, worms
Reproductive system – childbirth (helps to speed things up), cleansing, irregular periods, menstrual difficulties

Respiratory system – asthma, bronchitis, colds, coughs, fortify the lungs, laryngitis, phlegm, sore throat, tonsillitis, whooping cough
Skeletal system – arthritis, gout, rheumatism
The skin – boils, carbuncles, dandruff, dermatitis, hair loss, head lice, scalp tonic, sores, warts, wounds
Urinary system – antiseptic to the urinary system, cystitis

Other healing properties

Helps the body to fight disease & germs, rheumatism

Psychological / Emotional benefits

Concentration, depression, exhaustion, fear, indecision, low spirits, memory, mental blocks, strengthen the nerves, trauma

Karen Ashton
THE ESSENTIAL OILS GUIDE

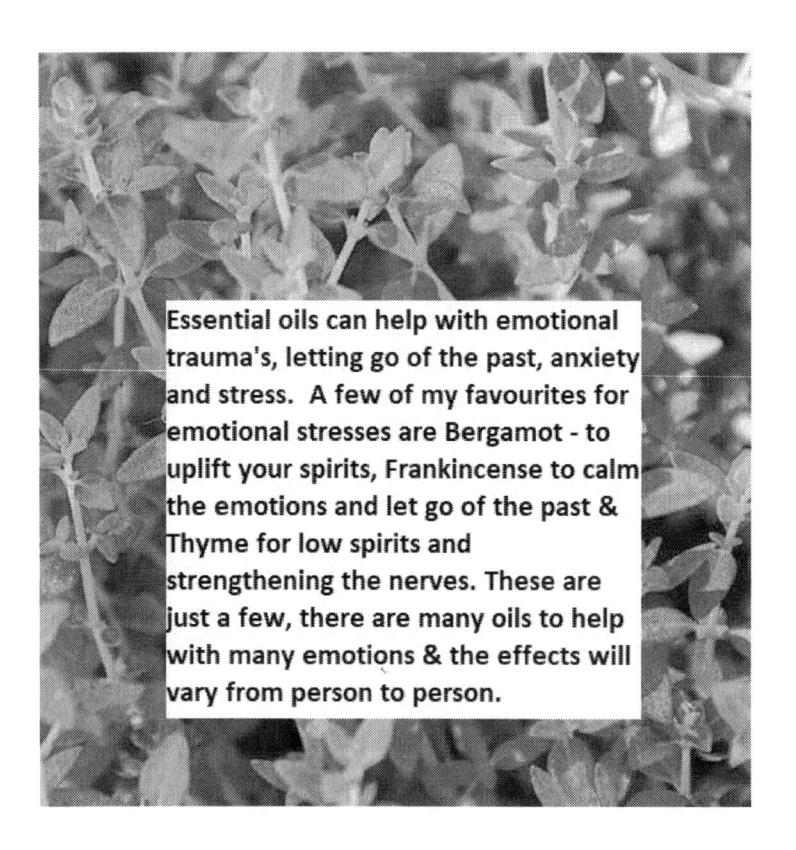

Essential oils can help with emotional trauma's, letting go of the past, anxiety and stress. A few of my favourites for emotional stresses are Bergamot - to uplift your spirits, Frankincense to calm the emotions and let go of the past & Thyme for low spirits and strengthening the nerves. These are just a few, there are many oils to help with many emotions & the effects will vary from person to person.

Karen Ashton
THE ESSENTIAL OILS GUIDE

Essential Oil Name

Vetivert

Image

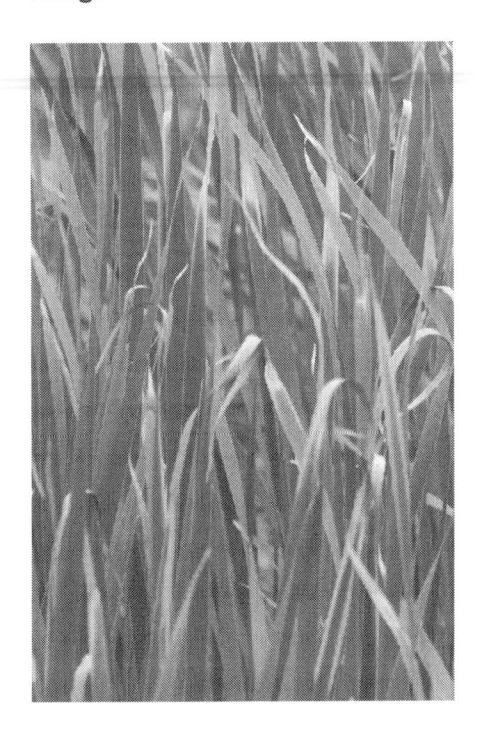

Botanical Name

Andropogon Muricatus

Plant

Grass / Root

Karen Ashton
THE ESSENTIAL OILS GUIDE

Plant Family

Gramineae

Category

Exotic

Note

Base

Objective

Balancing, Stress relief

Associated Planet

No known associated planet

Extraction Method

Distillation

Main chemical constituents

Acid, Alcohol, Aldehyde, Ketone, Sesquiterpene

Aroma

Deep, earthy, smoky

Karen Ashton
THE ESSENTIAL OILS GUIDE

Properties

Antiseptic, Aphrodisiac, Nervine, Sedative, Tonic

Contra-Indications / Precautions

- No known precautions

Benefits Body Systems

Circulatory system – blood flow, fortify red blood corpuscles
Nervous system – balancing on the central nervous system
Reproductive system – sexual problems, tonic to the reproductive system
Skeletal system – arthritis, rheumatism
The skin – Acne

Other healing properties

Helps to keep disease at bay, physical exhaustion, helps to restore the body back to health, insomnia, rheumatism

Psychological / Emotional benefits

Balancing, calming, centred, cleanses the aura, exhaustion, grounding, impatience, insecurity, mood

Karen Ashton
THE ESSENTIAL OILS GUIDE

swings, openness, panic, protection, psychological problems, restlessness, sensitivity, settles the nerves, stress, tension

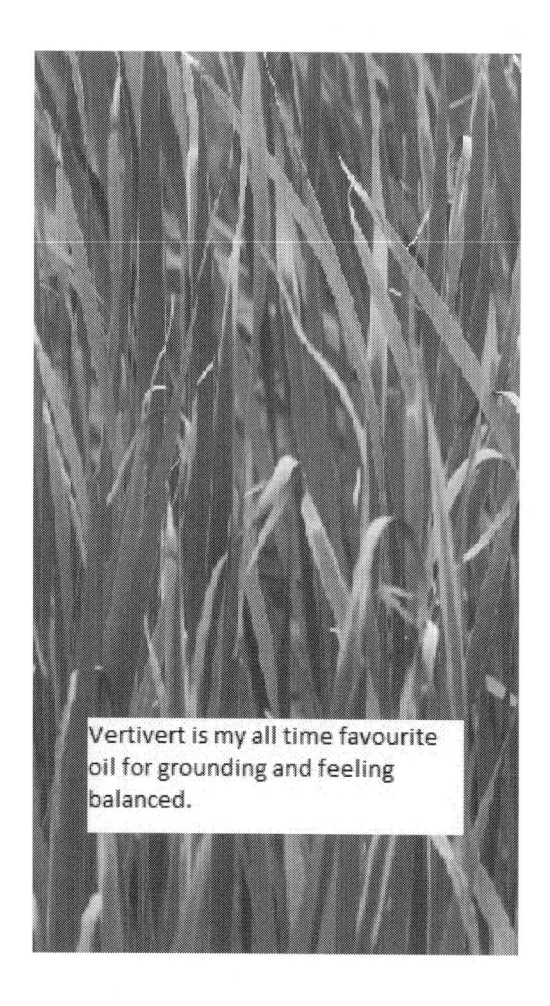

Vertivert is my all time favourite oil for grounding and feeling balanced.

Karen Ashton
THE ESSENTIAL OILS GUIDE

Essential Oil Name

Ylang Ylang

Image

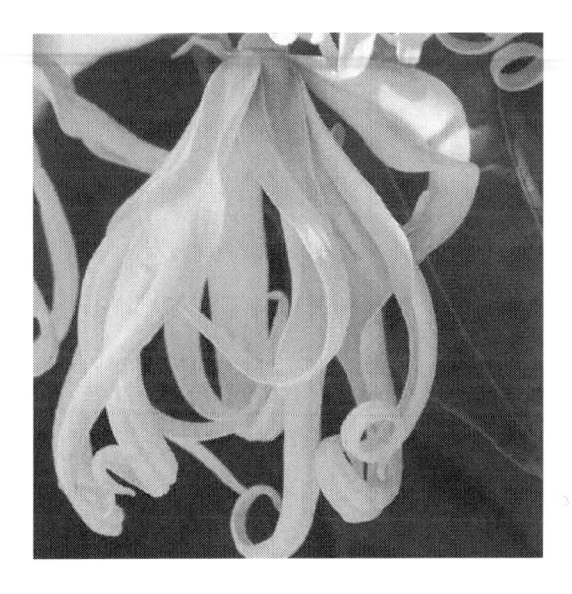

Botanical Name

Cananga odorata

Plant

Flowers

Karen Ashton
THE ESSENTIAL OILS GUIDE

Plant Family

Annonaceae

Category

Exotic

Note

Base

Objective

Relaxation

Associated Planet

Venus

Extraction Method

Distillation

Main chemical constituents

Acid, Alcohol, Ester, Eugenol, Farnesol, Geraniol, Phenol, Sesquiterpene, Terpene

Karen Ashton
THE ESSENTIAL OILS GUIDE

Aroma

Exotic, heavy & floral

Properties

Antidepressant, Antiseptic, Aphrodisiac, Hypotensive, Sedative

Contra-Indications / Precautions

- May cause headaches if used in excess
- Could cause irritation to sensitive skin

Benefits Body Systems

Circulatory system – heartbeat (rapid), high blood pressure
Digestive system – intestinal infections
Endocrine system – adrenal flow regulator, hormone balancing
Nervous system – relaxing on the nervous system
Reproductive system – frigidity, impotence, sexual problems, tonic to the womb
Respiratory system – rapid breathing
The skin – combination skin, dandruff, dry skin, hair growth, oily skin, scalp stimulant, sebum balancing, tonic

Karen Ashton
THE ESSENTIAL OILS GUIDE

Other healing properties

Jet lag

Psychological / Emotional benefits

Anger, anxiety, depression, fear, joy, frustration, guilt, impatience, insomnia, irritability, panic, sedative, self-control, shock

Karen Ashton
THE ESSENTIAL OILS GUIDE

Safety Guidelines

To avoid degradation, it is important to store the oils correctly. Here are some safety guidelines:

- ✓ Keep out of reach of unattended children, pets and anyone with special needs. Always ensure the integral dropper is in place as this acts as a guard against over consumption should the product fall into the wrong hands.
- ✓ Keep products away from delicate eye areas. If an accident occurs with neat essential oil flush the eyes with cold full fat milk or vegetable oil to dilute.
  If an accident occurs with diluted oil flush with clean warm water. If stinging is still present seek immediate medical advice.
- ✓ Keep products away from plastics, polished surfaces and all naked flames or sources of ignition.
- ✓ Do not take essential oils internally unless under strict medical supervision or if in consultation with an aromatherapist qualified to this level.
- ✓ Never use an undiluted essential oil directly on the skin. Always dilute in a suitable base product. Lavender and Tea Tree can be used

neat in very small amounts 1 – 2 drops but not on a regular basis.
- ✓ If you are pregnant, suffer from epilepsy, high/low blood pressure or any specific condition, please seek medical advice before using any aromatherapy products.
- ✓ Care must also be taken with certain oils (especially citrus oils) before exposure to direct sunlight to avoid photosensitivity.
- ✓ When adding essential oils to bath water dilute the oil first in a small amount of full fat milk or dispersing carrier oil. If neither is available be sure to agitate the water after adding the oil so it does not settle on the top of the water and cause irritation.
- ✓ Always mix the oil with water before burning in an oil burner. Never use undiluted!
- ✓ Try to regulate the use of any essential oil as constant use over time may in isolated cases cause sensitisation, nausea or headaches, and its therapeutic benefits may lessen.
- ✓ Certain oils may cause skin sensitivity or adverse reaction in some individuals. Discontinue use immediately if this occurs. If susceptible to this kind of reaction it is

always best to do a skin patch test before use on a larger area.
- ✓ Do not use machinery or drive a motor vehicle immediately following a relaxation treatment especially after using soporific oils, e.g. Clary Sage.
- ✓ Always work in a well-ventilated area.
- ✓ If working professionally with clients, In between use, air the treatment room and allow yourself a break of at least five minutes. Remember, you are inhaling & absorbing the oils too! Working in a well-ventilated room is advisable.
- ✓ If working professionally, always complete a detailed consultation to ascertain a client's physical and psychological condition, along with any medication they may be taking.
- ✓ Avoid prolonged use of the same essential oil as the therapeutic benefits may lessen.
- ✓ If you have hypersensitive skin it may be advisable to carry out a simple skin test before using the essential oil for the first time, by applying a small portion of the blended oil to a small area of skin first before applying all over or using in the bath.
- ✓ Never use an essential oil with which you are not familiar with.

Karen Ashton
THE ESSENTIAL OILS GUIDE

- ✓ Essential oils should be stored in dark amber glass bottles in normal to cool temperatures (approx. 65 Fahrenheit / 18 centigrade) with lids secured tightly to prevent evaporation.
- ✓ Wash hands thoroughly in between use to remove as much of the oil as possible.
- ✓ Store the oils away from direct sunlight
- ✓ Store the oils for the correct storage period – check manufacturers recommendations & shelf life
- ✓ Only use the essential oils for their correct use and dilution
- ✓ Ensure, when purchasing, that your products have undergone quality testing and constituent testing. An MSDS sheet should be available

Karen Ashton
THE ESSENTIAL OILS GUIDE

Objectives chart

(T) Top　　　(M) Middle　　　(B) Base

Relaxation	Uplift/ Stimulation	Balancing	Stress relief
Benzoin (B)	Basil (T)	Bergamot (T)	Basil (T)
Chamomile (M)	Eucalyptus (T)	Black Pepper (M)	Benzoin (B)
Cypress (M)	Fennel (M)	Cedarwood (B)	Bergamot (T)
Frankincense (B)	Ginger (B)	Clary Sage (M)	Cedarwood (B)
Jasmine (B)	Grapefruit (T)	Geranium (M)	Chamomile (M)
Lavender (M)	Mandarin (T)	Juniper (M)	Clary Sage (M)
Lavender Spike (T)	Tea Tree (T)	Lavandin (M)	Cypress (M)
Marjoram (M)	Thyme (T)	Lemon (T)	Frankincense (B)
Neroli (B)		Lemongrass (T)	Geranium (M)
Orange (T)		Myrrh (B)	Grapefruit (T)
Petitgrain (T)		Patchouli (B)	Jasmine (B)
Rosemary (M)		Peppermint (T)	Lavender (M)
Sandalwood (B)		Rose (B)	Lemongrass (T)
Ylang Ylang (B)		Rosemary (M)	Marjoram

Karen Ashton
THE ESSENTIAL OILS GUIDE

			(M)
		Vetivert (B)	Neroli (B)
			Patchouli (B)
			Petitgrain (T)
			Rose (B)
			Rosemary (M)
			Sandalwood (B)
			Vetivert (B)

Karen Ashton
THE ESSENTIAL OILS GUIDE

Skin type chart

(T) Top (M) Middle (B) Base

Combination	Dry	Mature	Oily	Sensitive
Frankincense (B)	Benzoin (B)	Benzoin (B)	Bergamot (T)	Chamomile (B)
Geranium (M)	Chamomile (M)	Cypress (M)	Cedarwood (B)	Jasmine (B)
Jasmine (B)	Jasmine (B)	Fennel (M)	Clary Sage (M)	Neroli (B)
Lavender (M)	Neroli (B)	Frankincense (B)	Cypress (M)	Rose (B)
Neroli (B)	Orange (T)	Neroli (B)	Fennel (M)	
Patchouli (B)	Patchouli (B)	Rose (B)	Frankincense (B)	
Rose (B)	Petitgrain (T)	Sandalwood (B)	Geranium (M)	
Ylang Ylang (B)	Rose (B)		Grapefruit (T)	
	Ylang Ylang (B)		Juniper (M)	
			Lemon (T)	
			Lemongrass (T)	
			Peppermint (T)	
			Petitgrain (T)	
			Rose (B)	
			Ylang Ylang (B)	

Karen Ashton
THE ESSENTIAL OILS GUIDE

Skin condition chart
(T) Top   (M) Middle   (B) Base

Acne	**Congestion**	**Dehydrated**	**Elasticity**
Basil (T)	Basil (T)	Cypress (M)	Benzoin (B)
Bergamot (T)	Fennel (M)	Sandalwood (B)	Chamomile (M)
Cedarwood (B)	Geranium (M)		Fennel (M)
Chamomile (M)	Grapefruit (T)		Jasmine (B)
Clary Sage (M)	Juniper (M)		Neroli (B)
Grapefruit (T)	Orange (T)		
Juniper (M)	Peppermint (T)		
Lavender (M)	Petitgrain (T)		
Lemongrass (T)	Rosemary (M)		
Orange (T)	Tea Tree (T)		
Patchouli (B)			
Petitgrain (T)			
Sandalwood (B)			
Vetivert (B)			

Karen Ashton
THE ESSENTIAL OILS GUIDE

Top, Middle, Base Note Chart

Top Note	Middle Note	Base Note
Basil	Black Pepper	Benzoin
Bergamot	Chamomile	Cedarwood
Eucalyptus	Clary Sage	Frankincense
Grapefruit	Cypress	Ginger
Lavender Spike	Geranium	Myrrh
Lemon	Juniper	Neroli
Lemongrass	Lavender	Patchouli
Mandarin	Lavandin	Rose
Orange	Marjoram	Sandalwood
Peppermint	Rosemary	Vetivert
Petitgrain		Ylang Ylang
Tea Tree		
Thyme		

You may see different views on which oils are top, middle or base notes, and some maybe both. i.e., Neroli is said to be a top or a base note depending on the other oils it is blended with. Ginger has been classed as a top note in other publications. Confused as to which category to put the oils in? Have a look at the descriptions of what a top, middle and a base note is, and how to tell the difference, then have a go at deciphering them yourself. What is a ginger essential oil to you? Is it a top, middle or a base?

Karen Ashton
THE ESSENTIAL OILS GUIDE

How my journey started

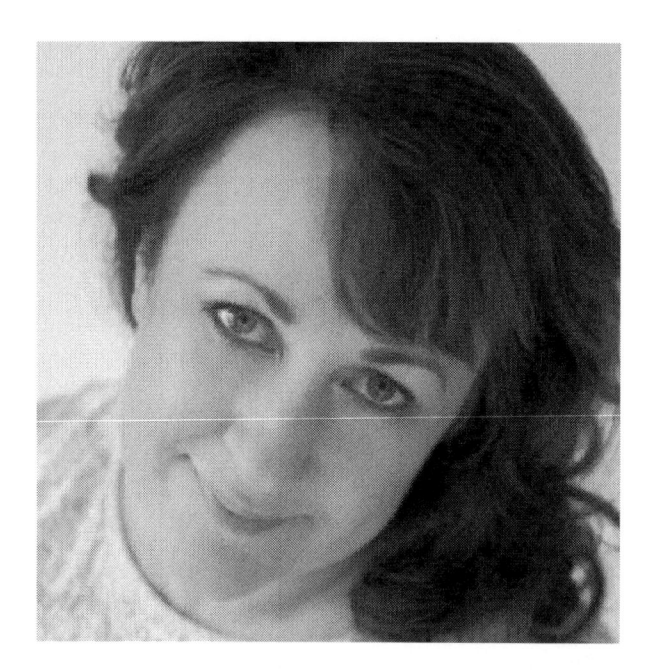

Karen Ashton

Back in 2003, a mum of 2 children under the age of 3, a wife and an office manager, life felt quite tough at this time and I needed something for 'me', I craved to feel independent and wanted to get my teeth stuck into something. So, my journey began with my love for aromatherapy. I wanted something I could do as a hobby but earn money out of at the same time, so I had this hair brain idea that I wanted to set up an online company selling essential oils and other aromatherapy-based

Karen Ashton
THE ESSENTIAL OILS GUIDE

products. To do this, I wanted to gain as much knowledge as I could on the oils before selling the products, so I enrolled on an aromatherapy course. Part of the course involved learning massage, now this may come as a surprise to some of you who know me, but I wasn't overly keen on the thought of massaging someone, despite this, I completed the course and I passed :-) I then decided to take the knowledge gained about the oils and use this, but I was unsure if I was going to use my massage skills again! ;-) Well, until a month or two later, when a few friends asked if they could have a massage, and after much debate, I decided, ok, I will. Well, being in my own surroundings, and creating a nice ambience in the room seemed to help a great deal, also knowing the client I was massaging seemed to help a little too. Afterwards, I thought, I can't be that bad, as I sent the client to sleep :-) Result! This wasn't so bad after all.

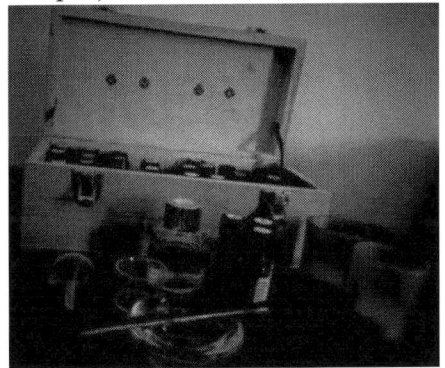

My online oil business was doing ok, Amber Oils, and my therapy business began, initially working

Karen Ashton
THE ESSENTIAL OILS GUIDE

from home, I started adding qualifications, reflexology, Indian head massage, and so on. I was really enjoying it by now. My business name became The Amber Retreat, and I even named and registered my house in Swindon, Wiltshire as this too. To progress the oil business, I looked into being able to blend my own oils and sell them, but this hit a wall, as I had to, back then, pay for each oil to be passed for manufacturing purposes, and this was going to set me back rather a lot of money, so this was put on hold.

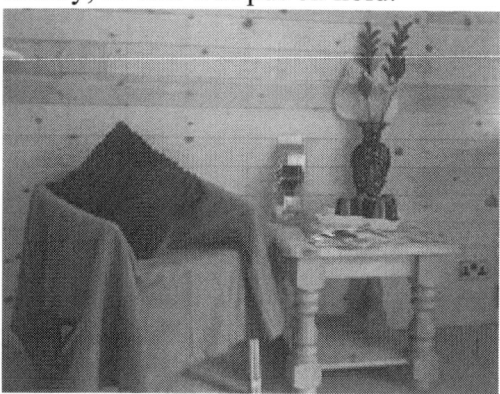

Karen Ashton
THE ESSENTIAL OILS GUIDE

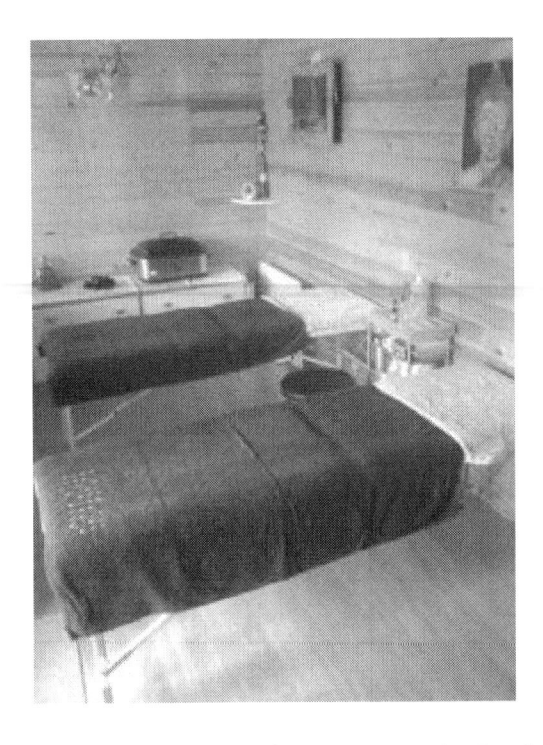

I continued, instead, to progress in the therapy side of my business. I decided I needed to build a client base and this would be really slow from home (Facebook and social media wasn't as widely used back then) so I wrote off to as many salons and hotels as possible to see if there were any rooms to rent on a part time basis (my boys were still pre-school at this stage so wanted the balance of looking after them too) Boom! I received 4 replies all wanting me to rent their room. I had to choose which one I wanted to go for. Anyway, I spent a few years, working at a couple different rooms at hair salons and back at home, in a cabin built in the garden, my dining room, a spare bedroom, even my lounge. I also went into business with a friend and we rented a spa within a hotel for 18 months, offering various therapies & managing staff. After many courses at various training centres, I started to run workshops and enrolled on a teacher training course at Cirencester college, this was when my next chapter started as I started to write course manuals and become an accredited training centre initially based in Swindon. I loved it! I had finally found my passion.

This was back in 2006 / 2007, & my marriage broke up during this year too, so I became a single mum to my 2 boys, who were then aged 5 & 6.

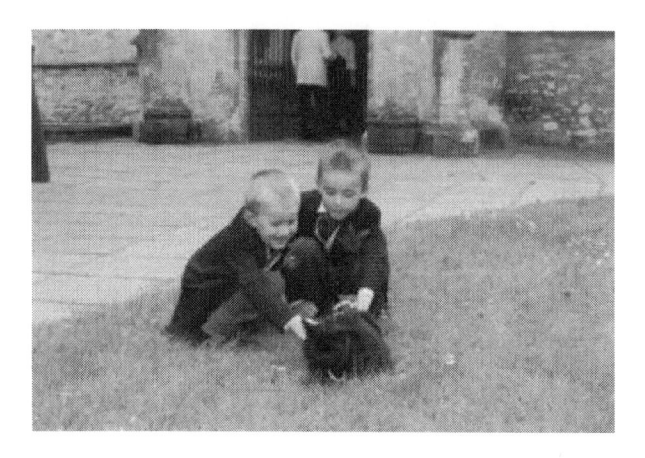

I then realised why I had the urge back in 2003 to become independent . . . I needed to support myself and my boys financially. My focus, to get me through this was setting up my training school.

Karen Ashton
THE ESSENTIAL OILS GUIDE

Teaching and passing on my skills and knowledge to others became my passion. As if that wasn't enough, in 2011 I decided a fresh start was in order for me and my boys, and the pull to move back to my roots, Bideford in North Devon was becoming bigger and bigger. When my 10 year old said to me one day, 'Mum it will be ok moving to Devon, because I will make lots of new friends, and I can still keep in touch with my old friends, my dad and family,' this was my catalyst I needed to get brave and 'feel that fear and just do it'. The house went on the market on 1st March 2011 and we had sold and moved into our new house in Bideford, by 3rd June 2011, I think the universe was telling me that this was the right thing to do :-)

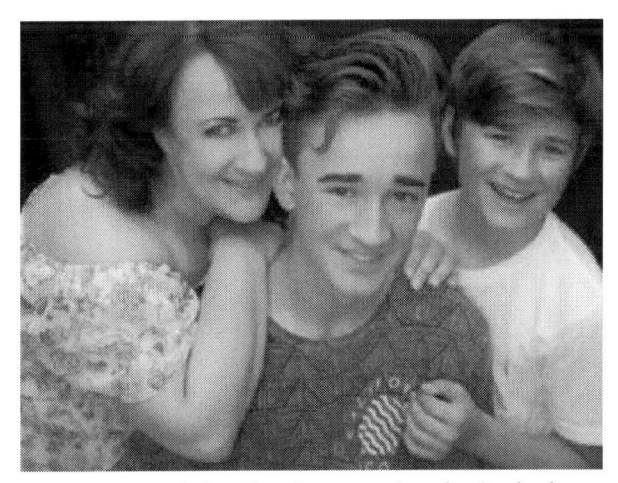

I kept my training business going in Swindon to give me the income to be able to move and start anew in Bideford. It took a couple of years to build the training up here while I continued to travel around the South West teaching in salons and spas, going where the demand took me. With the support of my wonderful parents, to help with my boys, this was what made this possible for me to do.

One of my biggest achievements was becoming a VTCT assessment, firstly in Swindon, secondly under the umbrella of a school in Gloucester, and then in South Molton, Devon. I have since become a sole registered centre for VTCT in my own right, in Bideford, Devon.

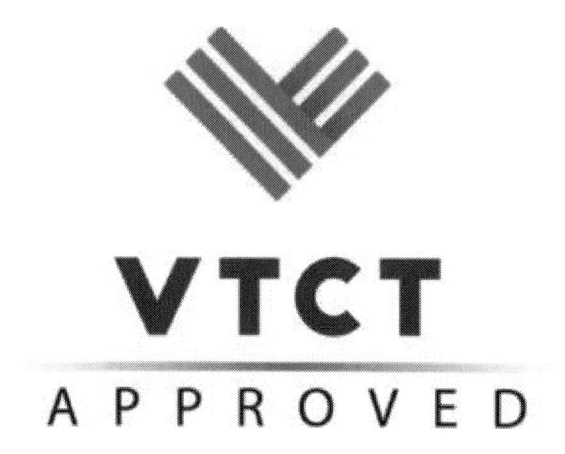

VTCT APPROVED

At the start of 2016, I met my soulmate, Jason. (What a way to start the new year)

Now, way back, I had 'placed an order with the universe for a man who knew how to massage,' well low and behold, one of the first things he told me about himself when I first met him, was he was massage and sports massage trained from 14 years ago. Yippee!! Thank you, universe, :-)

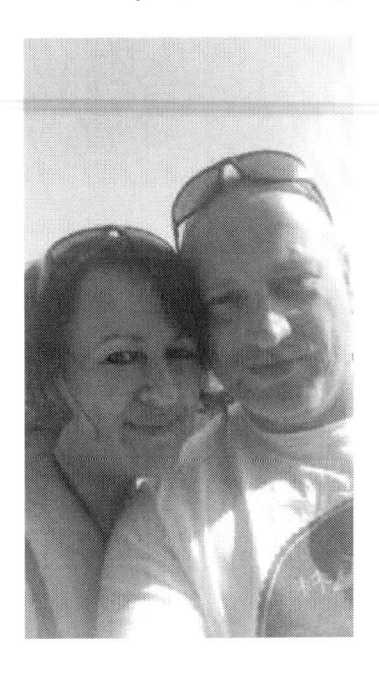

An emergency op in 2016, and personal needs of his son, put paid to his job and teaching as a martial arts instructor, for the time being, and I got brave, once more, and welcomed him into the business, to help me with sales & marketing & teaching in sports massage and other massage courses.

Karen Ashton
THE ESSENTIAL OILS GUIDE

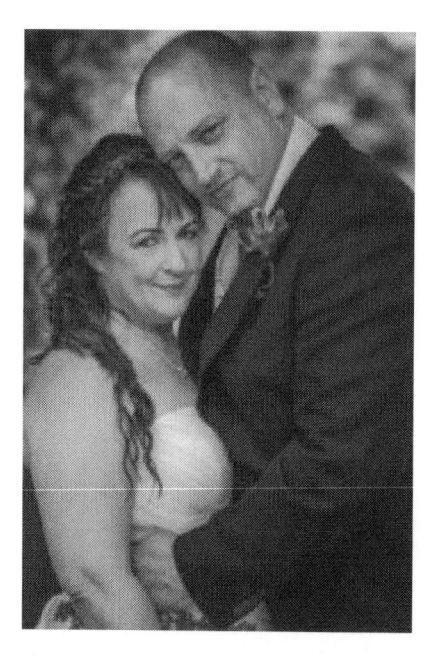

In August 2017, we married 🙂

In August 2017, I had welcomed my 3000th student through the doors of Holistic Therapies Training, and through the many years of ups and downs; blood, sweat and tears; sleepless nights and anxieties, I am still living my dream and loving the journey.

To be continued . . ..

Karen Ashton
THE ESSENTIAL OILS GUIDE

About the author

Karen is a fully qualified beauty and holistic therapist, assessor, verifier and teacher. She has many therapies 'under her belt' and is very passionate about her work. Karen has run her own therapy business since 2003 as well as professional training in beauty and holistic therapies and offers a range of professional training to therapists as well as people looking for career changes. She is dedicated to providing her students with the highest standards of education in beauty & holistic therapies. Holistic Therapies has always been an interest of hers and she is so pleased to be able to pass on her passion for such a wonderful profession. Karen is qualified in and teaches the following therapies: Aromatherapy (level 3 & 4), Baby Massage Instructor, Beauty therapy level 2, Body Massage (level 3 & 4), Body Wrap, Chinese Body Massage, Cognitive behavioural therapy, Cosmetic Tanning, Colour Therapy, Crystal Healing, Holistic Facial, Hopi Ear Candling, Hot Stones Massage, Indian Head Massage, Manual Lymphatic Drainage Massage, Make Up level 3, Nail technician, Oriental Face Massage, Oriental Hand Massage, Pregnancy Massage, Provide therapies for clients with cancer & other life limiting conditions level 4, Reflexology (level 3 & 4), Reiki 1, 2 & master, Sports Massage (Level 3 & 4), Stress Management level 4, Thai Foot Massage, City & Guilds in Further Education teaching level 4. VTCT Assessor level 3, IQA (verifiers) level 4.

Karen Ashton
THE ESSENTIAL OILS GUIDE

"Teaching is a passion of mine and I love to pass on my skills and knowledge to my students. I enjoy small group training as I feel the students can receive more of my attention throughout the day. I also love to teach students on a one to one basis as the training can be tailored specifically to the student and they can work to their own pace without feeling the pressure of keeping up with their fellow students. This method of teaching has proven very popular with my students as they can also book the training to suit their schedule, whether it be to fit around their current job or children, rather than booking a group course on a specific day. The training days are always fun & relaxed allowing the students to gain maximum knowledge and enjoyment out of the day. My students also receive ongoing mentoring from me whether in development of their skills or setting up and running their therapy business, I'm always on hand to answer any questions or give advice."

Holistic Therapies Training

www.holistictherapiestraining.co.uk

Karen Ashton
THE ESSENTIAL OILS GUIDE

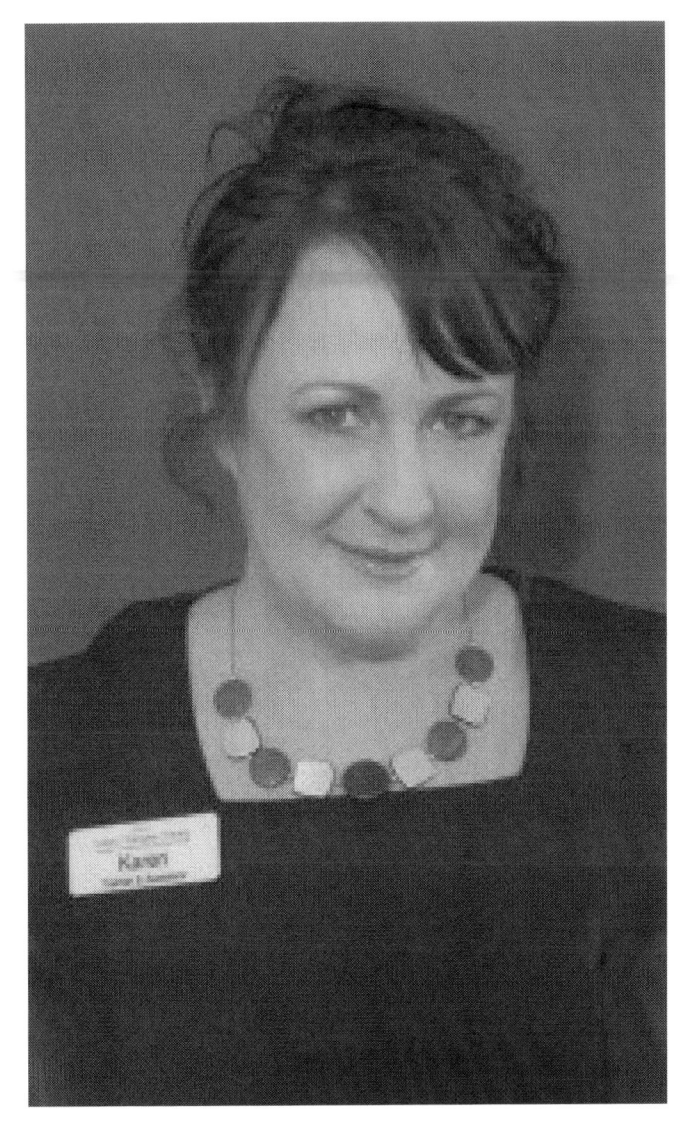

Thank you for reading!

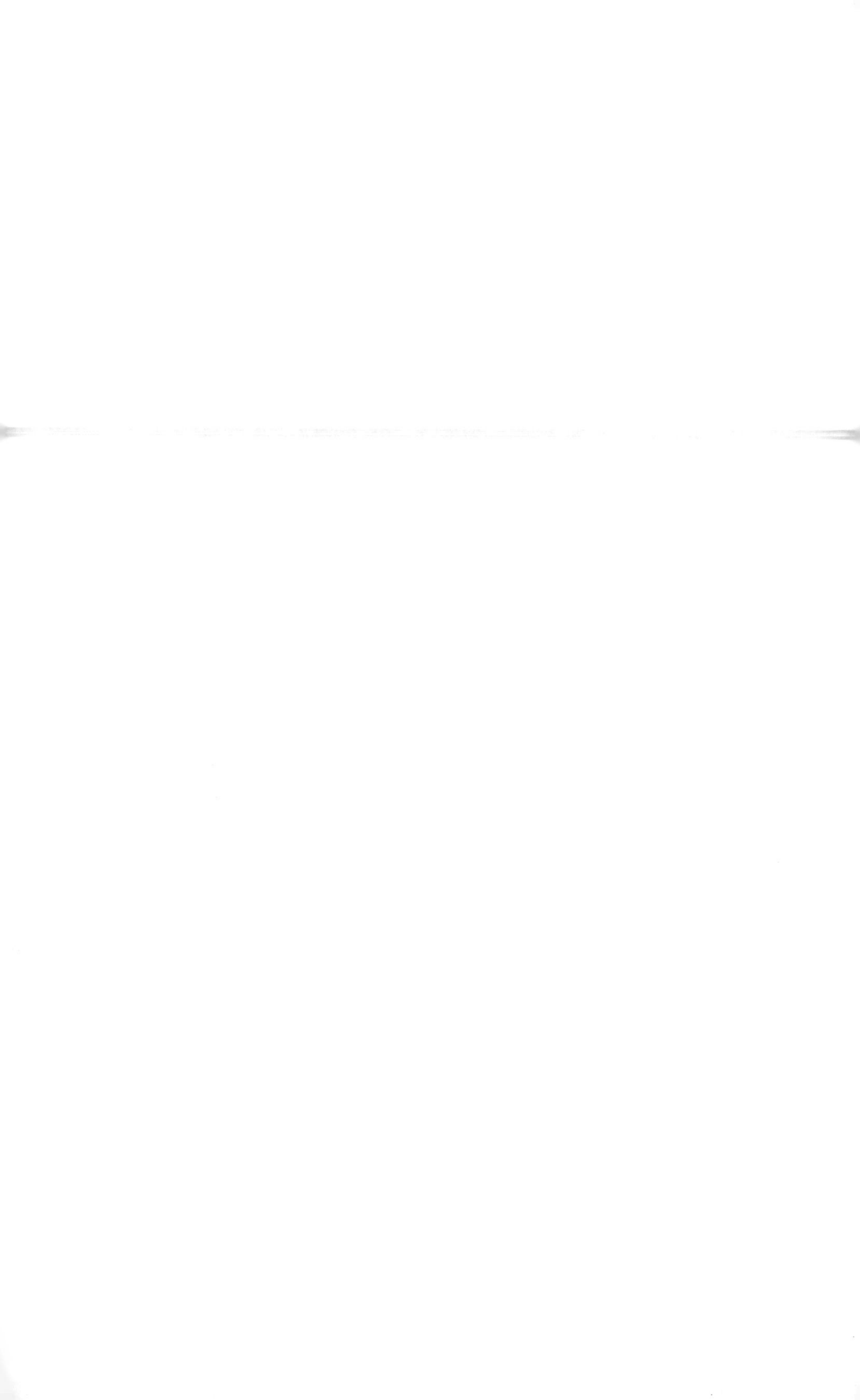

Printed in Great Britain
by Amazon